CHOOSE

TO BE

HEALTHY

DISCOVER HOW TO EMBRACE
LIFE AND LIVE FULLY

SUSAN SMITH JONES, PH.D.

FOREWORD BY DR. WAYNE W. DYER
PREFACE BY JOHN WOODEN

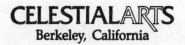
CELESTIALARTS
Berkeley, California

Celestial Arts
P.O. Box 7327
Berkeley, California 94707

Cover design by Ken Scott
Cover photo by Mark Farrell
Text design by Paul Reed
Typography by HMS Typography, Inc.

Library of Congress Cataloging-In-Publication Data

Jones, Susan Smith
    Choose to be healthy.

    Bibliography: p.
    1. Health.   2. Self-respect   3. Holistic medicine.
I. Title.
RA776.5.J565   1987   613   86-26842
ISBN 0-89087-482-4

Manufactured in the United States of America

First Printing, 1987

        4   5 — 91

TABLE OF CONTENTS

This book is lovingly dedicated to my mother, June, who by example has taught me to celebrate life and live fully

and

This book is dedicated to you, the reader—because you make a difference in the world. This book will renew your hope, inspire your soul, lift your spirits, make you think, and strengthen your resolve to live the life you've always wanted to live. You can be healthy and peaceful, and you can bring about a peaceful world. You are important to the well-being of planet Earth.

ACKNOWLEDGMENTS

My loving, heartfelt appreciation and gratitude to my Mom, for her eternal unconditional love, guidance and support; to my Dad, for his ever-presence and love; to Stormy, Golden, and Ralph for always being there; to Sylvia Arons, for being my mirror and steering me in the right direction; to Bryce B. Carr, for showing me how to be more childlike and to live more from my heart; to Lt. Warren Rigby, for giving me the gift of sunshine, the ocean and sea breeze; to Jesse Castañeda and Carolyn Murray, M.D., for being the greatest workout partners and for showing me the joy of friendship; to June, Jamie, Reid, Sparkie and Ad, Jackie, Fritzie and Benny, my family, for reminding me that what really matters in life can only be seen with the heart; to Rev. George Marks, for joining with me in embracing life and connecting in the Light; to Peter Zschalig, Hannah and Phil Krammer, James Lennon, Helen Guppy, Mark Ferrell, Elise Klysa, Wayne R. Bianchin, Rick McCoy, Rev. Bob Benedict and my special MacGYVER, for enriching the quality of my life; to the Ken and Barkley Company at KABC Radio in Los Angeles, for helping me through so many early morning workout sessions; to UCLA's Department of Cultural and Recreational Affairs, for giving me the opportunity of doing what I love to do for more than fifteen years; to my special friend, Paramahansa Yogananda, for his illuminating guidance, spiritual teachings and resplendent inspiration in my life; to Wayne Dyer, Ph.D., John Wooden, Leo Buscaglia, Eknath Easwaran, Ole Hendriksen, Peace Pilgrim, Mother Theresa, John R. Price, Paul Bragg, Jerry Jampolsky, Dr. Norman Walker, Dr. Herbert Shelton, Joy Gross, Ann Wigmore, Bernard Jensen, Roy Eugene Davis, Paavo Airola, Ph.D., Nathan Pritikin, Ralph Waldo Emerson, Henry David Thoreau, Eric Butterworth, Emmet Fox, A Course in Miracles, Norman Vincent Peale, O. Carl Simonton, M.D., Norman Cousins, Dennis Weaver, Buckminster Fuller, Captain Jacques Cousteau, and Dr. Masaharu Taniguchi for having a positive influence on my career and life; to Paul Reed and Celestial Arts Publishers for supporting my vision; and most especially to my very best friend and guiding Light, Jesus Christ, for joy and Love, for teaching me about forgiveness and peace, and for showing me how to embrace life, live fully and celebrate this gift of Divinity within us all.

PREFACE

When Susan asked me to write this preface, I was somewhat skeptical, but after being given the opportunity for an advance reading and taking advantage of that, I was delighted. For more that fifteen years she has been a fitness instructor at UCLA, motivating and inspiring students, staff, and faculty to become healthy and fit—and to celebrate life.

This book is informative and refreshing. While her exploration of "holistic" living isn't really new, she, nonetheless, has a special ability to take complex thoughts, research, and experience and to present it in a clear, practical, and engaging manner. What I really appreciate about Susan is her ability to articulate feelings and describe experiences that all of us have had in a way that allows us to understand our own challenges, to make clearer who and what we are as Divine beings, and how we can live our highest potential. Susan explores the elements necessary to create a life that is filled with positive choices and positive results. She shows us how health and happiness are so much more than just feeling fine, but are, as she writes in the first chapter, "...body, mind, and spirit working as one—harmoniously." This happens, she says, as a direct result of the choices we make in life—how we eat, exercise, think, play, and rest. Yes, it is true that the choices we make in life and our ability to keep all things in proper perspective are what make us.

For many years now, in my coaching, writing, and lectures, I have talked about my "pyramid to success" and how each of us must take responsibility for our lives and how we can all enrich the quality of life on this planet by how we choose to live our lives. Susan conveys this message with love and a sincere desire to assist you in creating your life beyond your highest dreams. She has done an outstanding job of telling you how to live a balanced life. I was impressed with how Susan tied together the physical, mental, emotional, and spiritual nature of life to provide a holistic approach to successful living. She has great insight and the world will be a better and more knowledgeable place because of her commitment to teaching the truth about health and living fully. Since I am a firm believer that *love* and *balance* are the most important essentials for a good life, I found this underlying thought very meaningful.

This is one of the most complete books I have read on how to be healthy, happy, and fully alive. I recommend it to anyone who wants to be healthier, happier, and more at peace with themselves and who wants to make a difference in this world. I know the thousands of people all over the world who love Susan and whose lives have been enhanced by her message are eagerly looking forward to this new book. They have a treat in store. In clear and beautiful prose, Susan tells us that health and peace are a conscious choice. And reading this book is a vital step in making that choice.

—John Wooden, UCLA (Ret.)

FOREWORD

by Dr. Wayne W. Dyer

I have long subscribed to the idea that all of life is a choice. When we let ourselves ultimately come to believe in the power of BEING a "choice-making" human being, we at last begin to take total responsibility for ourselves and our unique destinies. Susan Jones provides us with a beautifully useful elaboration on this theme of choosing our own greatness in virtually all life areas. She has taken great pains to provide extremely valuable information on how to take total control of ourselves, by first and foremost taking responsibility for the quality of the journey that we call life.

In simple, easy-to-read and (most importantly) easy-to-apply language, this book outlines an approach to living that is possible for every single reader to achieve, if they are willing to make it happen for themselves. Regardless of your current state of physical or emotional disrepair, you can take this book, read carefully, and begin now to *Choose to Be Healthy*.

A very strong thread of spirituality and "higher consciousness thinking" is woven throughout the pages of this book. Susan cannot help but write from this perspective, because I know her to be a respecter of the divine forces operating ubiquitously in each and every one of us. Susan believes strongly in the importance of love in each one of our lives. Not the kind of love that requires a partner in order to be fulfilled, but the divine love that is itself the harmony that holds every living cell together. Without the internal harmony in a cell, it will attack and attempt to devour the cell adjacent to itself, and ultimately will destroy the entire organism. So it is with divine love. Each of us is a cell in the body called humanity. When we have harmony within, we cooperate with the cells next to us, and when this harmony or love is missing, we fight our adjacent cells, leading to destruction of the totality of all of humanity. As we fight anything, we become weaker, for in so doing we are violating the very principle that holds the universe together. That is harmony and cooperation. You will see Susan's enormous regard for this spiritual (not necessarily religious, but spiritual) force that guides the universe, and each life form that occupies its own unique place in this perfect universe.

Recent efforts by chemists and other scientists have produced a synthetic form of wheat, that looks, tastes, smells, feels and acts like wheat. To the naked eye it appears that this product is definitely wheat. However, when placed in the ground, something quite strange happens that sets it apart from authentic wheat. It will not grow! Despite its appearance and nutritional make-up, synthetic wheat will not grow and reproduce naturally. Why? What is missing? The absent ingredient is the "life-force" that can never be reproduced synthetically. So it is with each of us. We need the "higher elements," whatever they may be, in order to grow as human beings. Susan, in these pages of her latest book, offers you a life plan that incorporates the authentic ingredients for choosing to be healthy, happy, and fully alive. She sprinkles her writing with marvelous quotations from the masters, both historic and contemporary, all of whom have made their own unique contributions to the betterment of mankind. Her writing is concise and useful, and the subject matter is universal. That being the improvement of the quality of life for all of us, and to help you, the reader, to forget about synthetic happiness, artificial health and phony fulfillment, and to replace them with a genuine, life-enhancing formula that will not only help you feel better, but to grow and flourish just like *real wheat* does when placed in a natural setting.

Everything we experience is a choice. Our personalities are the result of the choices we make. Our level of fitness is a result of those same opportunities to choose to be healthy. Our emotional condition likewise is a consequence of our choices. And when you really consider this concept of choice, it boils down to the way that we choose to *think*. We become what we think about all day long. Thus, our personality, state of health, and our emotional stability all revolve around thinking. Learn to think healthy, to visualize yourself as a success, and eventually your actions will follow those internal self-pictures. It can be no other way. Our thinking is our mental practice, just like hitting a backhand a thousand times is our physical practice. With enough practice you will achieve what you desire. That is how thought works.

Susan's approach is to help you to see that you are important enough to seek your own full measure of happiness and success, and that you are divine enough, just by the nature of your existence, to be heard. As you read through the pages of this powerful book, remind yourself that you are indeed divine enough to be answered. Think of a puzzle with one piece missing and realize that the entire picture is incomplete without that one piece. Then see yourself as one piece in this entire picture called humanity, and that the whole thing is incomplete without you. That is how important you are. Your completeness makes us all whole, and Susan's fine book will help you not only to grasp this notion, but to take action, beginning now, to correct any self-imposed limits you may have placed on yourself.

— *Dr. Wayne W. Dyer*
Author of:
Your Erroneous Zones
Pulling Your Own Strings
The Sky's the Limit
Gifts from Eykis
What Do You Really Want for
  Your Children
You'll See It When
  You Believe It

INTRODUCTION

You might look at this book as my personal journal that I've chosen to reveal to you. Over the years my life and experience of being in this world has changed in many ways.

As long as I can remember, I have always enjoyed writing. It has been a hobby, a form of therapy and self-healing that has been a large part of my working life. Through writing I have come to understand my life with more clarity and to appreciate the wisdom from the lessons that life presents to me. By expressing my thoughts and feelings on paper, I've found clues, direction, and answers to help take care of unfinished business or unresolved conflict.

Because for me it is more lucid than thinking or talking, writing assists me in identifying the petty and troubling beliefs that keep me from being all I was created to be.

Lessons are more useful if they are shared with others, so I am grateful to have this opportunity to share some of my life with you. I hope that by reading about my journey, your life will be enriched.

Henry David Thoreau once said, "The mass of men lead lives of quiet desperation." I hope that by reading and *participating* in this book, your life will become a magnificent adventure. Active participation is important in reading this book. It's not what we read that makes a difference in our lives. Rather, it's how we apply and experience the material that is of real value. At the end of each chapter you'll find Self-Discovery Questions and Action Choices for you to complete. Don't pass over these. Take time with each item. No one has to see what you've written. This should be your personal transformation workbook. This special section will assist you in getting to know yourself better. And, after all, isn't that the key ingredient to living to your fullest potential?

Right now you have the power and ability to transform and enrich the quality of your life and life on this planet. You can choose to glow in high self-esteem and radiate strength. No one has ever stopped you but you. You can be all you were meant to be—healthy, happy, successful, prosperous, and at peace. You can live and be your vision. But it requires that you make a conscious choice to do so. This moment—right now—can be a new beginning. No longer need you repeat the past, worry about the future, or struggle through life as a victim of circumstance. For as you live your life today—absorbed in the present moment, letting your heart light shine, being responsible and accountable for who you are and what you want to become—you will come to experience a life more splendid, more wondrous, and more magical than you ever dreamed possible.

You see, all the responsibility is on your shoulders. You cannot blame something or someone outside yourself for your own failure to live your vision. It's simply a matter of choice. Choose to be healthy and choose to be peaceful—and your world will be enlightened.

Of course, I didn't wake up one morning and find that my life had simply turned around. For a long time I was very confused. I had many questions that needed answers, and I discovered through countless struggles that the answers cannot be found in the outside world. Like most of you, I was taught to seek answers *outside* myself—in school, magazines, books, from experts, or from the stars. Yes, these sources have their place. But the answers to the really important questions—the spiritual ones—can be found only by turning inward. Life is within each of us. By looking within we will find that we are never alone. And we are the gift and miracle we've been seeking. When we start living fully, we inspire excellence in all who share our lives.

What I have found happening in my life is that as I gradually develop a more quiet and clear awareness, my living habits naturally come into harmony with my total environment, with my past involvements, present interests, and future priorities. When you are in touch with your innermost Self, when you begin to discover who you truly are, and when you choose to commit to live from inner guidance rather than play the victim of the world you see, the changes in your life will come naturally.

There is so much more to health than a strong body and a clear mind. Being healthy implies a harmonious balance between one's physical, emotional, mental, and spiritual selves and a recognition that these are not separate. We are a whole being created in the image and likeness of God.

Henry David Thoreau once said, "How prompt we are to satisfy the hunger and thirst of our bodies; how slow to satisfy the hunger and thirst of our souls." Don't consider your body a lump of flesh, but rather a noble instrument; within is the source of all power. All we have to do is tap into it. Wisdom, light, and love are within each of us and make up the ribbon that unites us all together.

I believe that all endeavors toward attaining better health are futile unless the healthy body is seen and used as the temple of God in which God's spirit dwells. Because of my belief, my emphasis is on physical exercise, proper diet, high thinking, and simple living. The body reflects the mind, and the mind reflects the spirit; hence the motivation to attain better health. This is what's right and true for me.

Finally, I believe that your choice to be healthy can also enrich the quality of life on planet Earth. For at one level we are all connected; each person is a wave in this ocean of life. When you choose to be a responsible, loving, forgiving, healthy, and happy person, living from integrity and oneness, this has a positive influence around the world, adding to the light. By the same token, choosing the opposite decreases light and wholeness. Each of us makes a difference in this tapestry of life by how we live. Become responsible, let go, surrender to living from your heart, the power within you, and as you do, so greater world harmony will be created. As a result, your experience of living will become magical and fulfilling and you will know what it means to be living the way you were created to be. Life will become an adventure, filled with celebration and joy. Wisdom, love, and light will be your constant companions. You will know peace. You will become peace itself. It's your choice. Choose to be healthy.

To laugh often and much; to win the respect of intelligent people and the affection of children; to earn the appreciation of honest critics and endure the betrayal of false friends; to appreciate beauty; to find the best in others; to leave the world a bit better, whether by a healthy child, a garden patch or a redeemed social condition; to know even one life has breathed easier because you have lived. This is to have succeeded.

—Ralph Waldo Emerson

If one advances confidently in the direction of his dreams, and endeavors to live the life which he has imagined, he will meet with success unexpected in common hours. He will put some things behind, will pass an invisible boundary; new, universal and more liberal laws will begin to establish themselves around and within him, or old laws will be expanded and interpreted in his favor in a more liberal sense, and he will live with license of a high order of beings.

—Henry David Thoreau

CHAPTER 1

CHOOSE TO

LIVE FULLY AND CELEBRATE LIFE

Hello,

I am fortunate and grateful to have this opportunity to spend time with you, sharing my life and thoughts in a way that I hope communicates and reflects the love I have for life. I see this as a voyage we'll take together, an adventure of hope, renewal, rejoicing, and making choices. Together we can create a healthy, peaceful, and magnificent world. You do make a difference. There is no one like you in this entire world, no one with your talents, your eyes and heart, with your fingerprints, your dreams. You are unique and have been given the power and ability to make your life, and this world, any way you want it to be. It doesn't matter where you've been, what you've done in the past, where you were born, how many mistakes you've made, or how old you are. Right now, right this moment, you can choose differently. You can choose to be all that you were created to be—healthy, happy, successful and, peaceful. You can feel totally alive, filled with celebration for life, the way you felt when you were a small child. Aliveness! It's a choice and it's your divine right. As we spend some time together through these pages, you will discover some of the ways I choose to live healthfully and what I think health is all about. You will find out that it's more than just feeling fine physically. So right now, choose to be healthy.

1

Wellness. Healthfulness. Aliveness. What do these words mean
to you? Take a moment now to close your eyes and think about some
time in your life when you felt at peace with yourself, excited about
your life, vibrant, and energetic.

For me wellness, healthfulness, or aliveness is allowing that state
of being to be yours every day, allowing your mind, body, and spirit
to work in harmony. It is being so filled with health and aliveness
that there is no room for anything else. It is much more than just
the absence of disease. It is a quality of life, a joy in living such that
every day, every moment, is a celebration. It is also about appreciating, respecting, nurturing, and loving our bodies and ourselves completely and unconditionally, which means giving up the ways we
treat ourselves lovelessly. Health is our natural state of being. Be true
to the truth about you. Be true to yourself and live fully.

Ralph Waldo Emerson said it so beautifully. "Health is your
greatest wealth." How true that is! Is your health an important part
of your life? Or do you assume that because nothing is really wrong
with you, that you don't need to make any positive changes in your
way of life? If you don't make time for health by making conscious
choices, you will have to take time for sickness.

This book really began about seventeen years ago—by accident,
so to speak. I was involved in a car wreck in which my back was
fractured. The diagnosis from the physician was that I would never
be able to carry anything heavier than a small purse, I would live
a lifetime of pain, and my fitness program would be a thing of the
past. This pronouncement was devastating. Helen Keller once said,
"When one door closes, another opens; but often we look so long
at the closed door that we do not see the one which has opened
for us."

After the accident all I could see was a closed door. I was filled
with depression, self-pity, confusion, and feelings of being vic-
timized. After a couple of weeks, I went to a favorite spot overlook-
ing the Pacific Ocean, where I often go when in need of inspiration.
And I had a heart-to-heart talk with my Self. I was convinced that
life was meant to be a magnificent adventure—to be lived joyfully,
peacefully, and healthfully. I was also clear that living my life the

way the doctor told me I would didn't align with my beliefs and desires. I just couldn't accept it. I knew I had a choice to make. And I did. Although I didn't know exactly how I could change my physical condition, I knew that there was a higher power within me that had the answers. And so I simply made a commitment to let go, to live from inner guidance, and to accept only vibrant, radiant health. Of course, it hasn't always been an easy road, and I have made many mistakes. Nonetheless, in retrospect I can see that the car accident was a wonderful, valuable experience, and it was out of my hitting a real low spot that my life turned around. Someone once said, "The darker the sky, the brighter the stars." It wasn't until I made a real commitment that amazing, and what some people would call miraculous, things began to come my way. I discovered the power of hope and faith—faith meaning sometimes having to believe when common sense tells you not to. I also discovered the power of commitment.

> Until one is committed there is hesitancy, the chance to draw back, always ineffectiveness. Concerning all acts of initiative and creation there is one elementary truth, the ignorance of which kills countless ideas and splendid plans: that the moment one definitely commits oneself, then providence moves too. All sorts of things occur to help one that would otherwise never have occurred. A whole stream of events issues from the decision, raising in one's favor all manner of unforeseen incidents and meetings and material assistance, which no man could have dreamt would have come his way.
>
> Are you in earnest? Seize this very minute. Whatever you can do, or dream you can...begin it. Boldness has genius, power and magic in it. Only engage and then the mind grows heated; begin and then the work will be complete.
>
> —Goethe

After my experience by the ocean, a whole stream of events began that assisted me in healing my condition. I found perfect books and magazines, heard exactly right tapes and lectures, and met people who told me about the correct foods, visualizations and meditations—much of which sounded weird to me at the time. During those months following the accident (and still to this day),

I made changes in my way of life, behavior, thoughts, and attitude. After examining me at my six-month checkup, the doctor shook his head in bewilderment, saying, "This just can't be. There is no sign of the fracture, you are free of pain, and you seem to be in perfect health. It's just miraculous." Perhaps it was; I've since discovered that miracles are a natural part of committing to wellness, peace, and living fully.

Each year since that event I have continued to grow—learning new ways to become healthier, to embrace the fullness of life, to be more open to living up to my highest potential. Through it all I've come to recognize the importance of choosing to be healthy, and to see how health, or lack thereof, affects every area of our lives.

As a result of the accident, I started thinking of my body differently. I began to see it as the temple of my spirit, the place where I lived, the vehicle for my expression. As Aristotle said, "Wherever I go, there I am." Because the body reflects the mind and the mind reflects the spirit, you must choose to make your body's health a top priority in your life.

Two years ago a man came to see me. He was and still is the president of a major corporation in America. He was impatient, aggressive, sometimes hostile, and unaware of how to make choices to support his well-being. He routinely put in six or seven 15-hour pressure-packed days a week at the office or traveling. He always had to be first, always had to be right, and always had to be busy with work to feel worthwhile. As a fancier of rich foods, he put away vast quantities of cheese, ice cream, steak, butter, processed foods and cream sauces. A typical breakfast would be his favorite sausage, which was composed of pork, pork liver, white rice, and hot spices—this he consumed with eggs, ham, and two cups of coffee. He knew his food was loaded with cholesterol and fat, but loved it all the same. His exercise was shifting gears in one of his expensive sports cars.

He was usually tired and thought his hot tub and a drink were all he needed to relax. It wasn't until he began to sink into a depression that his wife encouraged him to have a checkup, his first in more than five years. Then came the shocker. This forty-year-old man discovered he had high blood pressure, and hardening of the arteries, and was told that if he didn't make some changes in his way of life immediately, he was headed for a heart attack within six months. It was also suggested that he have quadruple heart bypass surgery.

As Providence would have it, the following day a friend of his who had heard about the doctor's prognosis recommended that he follow the program outlined in my series of seven (7) audiocassettes, *Celebrate Life!* That's how we met. We worked together on his Wellness Program. His experiences and adventures over these past twenty-four months have been a great inspiration to me, for I had never worked with anyone who was so stressed, so unhealthy, and who led such an unhealthy way of life. During our first visit he made a choice—and he chose to make a commitment to changing his life and to being healthy. Today both he and his family are the picture of health. Recently, the family participated together in a 10K run and left the following day on a two-week health and fitness vacation.

Be aware that when you truly commit to something, be it better health, better relationships, prosperity, or peacefulness, when with your mind, body, heart, and soul you want to change something, patterns unlike your goal will come up for you to own, acknowledge, understand, and release. At that point it may seem easier to slip back into those more familiar patterns. Don't. And sometimes, in spite of your burning commitment, things look like they're getting worse for you. This has happened to me many times. I remember right after my car accident and making a commitment to vibrant health, I saw any sign of recovery seem to slip right down the drain as the pain and struggle seemed to get worse with each passing day. But it does begin to change. You'll become stronger and will acquire awareness and understanding from your weaknesses and will grow from them. Building a strong foundation is essential to lasting aliveness. If you choose the old, familiar course, you remain tied to your past and to your weaknesses, and are thus unable to correct them or to play up your strengths.

Similarly, as I've committed to better relationships in my life, I've seen some take a turn for the worse before they got better, as well as some that dissolved altogether. As I became more comfortable with that, I understood that when I ask for something, oftentimes what I have now may have to disappear to make room for what I want. One of the keys to softening our transitions in life is our ability to focus, to pay attention. No matter what comes up, no matter how off-course your life may seem, continue, with every fiber of your being, to pay attention and stay focused on what you want. Staying focused is a powerful tool and can determine your experiences in life. Full attention costs no money, but requires discipline and training. Strive toward being clearly focused with full attention—the intentional channeling of awareness—as much as possible in everything you do. Choose to focus only on life-affirming things, and take your attention off anything unlike that.

Collectively, this country has been making some poor choices. Any night turn on the TV and look at the kinds of commercials they have, or flip open any woman's magazine and look at the advertisements. Everywhere we look, we are bombarded with the notion that there's something to take for every ailment, whether it's a headache, constipation, fatigue, sleeplessness, body odor, hemorrhoids, diarrhea, indigestion, or bad breath. We buy into these ads and believe that we must put our faith in something outside the body in order to get better. We have forgotten how wonderfully capable our body really is, how efficient it is in taking care of itself, if we first make some conscious, wholesome choices.

I've got some news that might be pretty astonishing to you. It's normal to be able to go to sleep at night without taking a pill. It's normal not to have headaches, sinus problems, indigestion, or shaky hands. It's normal to be truly well. But we must first get out of our own way and support this magnificent body in what it needs to function optimally and fully. It's simply a matter of choice. Being healthy and living fully comes from making a commitment and choosing to be all you are capable of being and assisting others in their journey. When you start choosing to live and be that way, life will come alive, will take on new meaning. Start now.

Right this moment, stop reading and think about how truly remarkable your body is. Buckminster Fuller told us that ninety-nine percent of who we are is invisible, untouchable, and unsmellable. The remaining one percent, the body in which you live, is absolutely exquisite. It is a miracle, yet so often taken for granted.

Cherish, appreciate, and nurture your body, for this is the first step to experiencing vibrant, radiant health. Start today and tune in more to your body. It is an incredible feedback machine. If you listen, you will discover that it actually talks to you. When you get a headache, for instance, your body is trying to tell you something. Listen to your body and be willing to deal with its communication. The key here is your willingness.

I believe that the body is truly a miracle of miracles, one to a customer, and should be highly respected, loved, and appreciated. The nutritionist and philosopher Paul Bragg has given us a vivid description of how wonderful the body really is in the following statement: "Now stop and think! The creator has presented you with the world's most wonderful machine—your own body. This miracle machine has its own non-stop motor (the heart), its own fueling system (the digestive tract), its own filtration system (the kidneys), its own temperature controls (the sweat glands), and so on. Indeed, this most remarkable contrivance even has the power to reproduce itself."

Clearly, this body of ours didn't happen by chance. It has been intricately designed and balanced as a complex physical, mental, and spiritual entity. That is to say, physically—you are what you eat and how you exercise; mentally—you are what you think; spiritually—you are what you believe. The key here is balance. Actually, wellness is no more than a delicate, harmonious balance. Plato said, "Health is a love affair between all the organs of the body," to which I would add, "and the mind and the spirit."

To experience total aliveness, don't let your health take a back seat to anything. If you have discovered an ailment, or you don't feel comfortable and confident with the way you look or feel, it affects every part of your life. It's as though you are looking at the world through cloudy eyes. Poor health interferes with relationships, business, family harmony, peace of mind—everything in your life.

So clear your eyes and begin to set some priorities. The wonderful thing about wellness is that you can choose to do something about it. You cannot blame your family, friends, doctors, environment, and so on, for how you feel and look. You must start to take responsibility for your own health. In fact, *healthfulness is simply a matter of choice.* Fortunately, it is always your choice.

Our lives are made up of perpetual choices. Moment to moment, we are always choosing. What we are consists of choosing what we think, what we imagine, how we react, what we eat, what we say, what we feel, and what we expect. When you reflect on it, it's fantastic. We have the freedom to create our lives and our world so that they are any way we want them to be. This choice has always been available—but now we must deliberately, consciously choose. We must each take back the responsibility for our own lives and start using the power that is ours to create what we want.

Where it starts is right where you are. It begins with how you feel about yourself—your self-image. Self-image is crucial in determining the quality of our lives. Whether we succeed or fail, enjoy our life or struggle—all depends on our self-image. In fact, numerous studies have concluded that our view of ourselves is the key factor in taking control of our lives. Develop a loving relationship, a warm friendship with yourself. It is out of that friendship that all your other relationships form. Stop being critical, judgmental, and unforgiving of yourself. When you are not feeling good about you, it creates a feeling of separateness from others. Also, notice what you criticize in others, for it is often that same characteristic that you are critical of in yourself. Others are our mirrors, reflecting ourselves back to us. Others also treat us how we've taught them to treat us. So really, *the only relationship you ever have to work on is your relationship with yourself.* It all starts with you. You can't celebrate another or expect others to celebrate you until you first celebrate yourself. Treat yourself with dignity. Honor the love inside you and everyone else. Keep your agreements with yourself. See yourself as a winner, because you truly are. In short, the better you feel about yourself, the better the rest of the world will look and be.

When you see yourself as a failure, you create a self-fulfilling prophecy. You attract to yourself that which you express. Your negative thoughts and attitude about yourself, whether they originated with your own self or with others, create beliefs that convince you of your inability to succeed. Because of this negative self-image, you feel unworthy and undeserving. If you feel you don't deserve success, don't deserve prosperity, don't deserve to enjoy life, don't deserve happy relationships, you settle for less than that to which you are entitled. When you feel unworthy, you cut yourself off from the fullness of life—peace, joy, love, harmony, prosperity, and health.

What is needed to disconnect this vicious cycle is to first love and accept ourselves, unconditionally. We have the capacity to become larger than the circumstances of our lives. Follow the advice of William James: "The most important thing in life is to live your life for something more important than your life." Next we must step beyond our limited beliefs and the beliefs of others that we have accepted as our own, and realize our importance to ourselves and to the world. Understand that you always did your best at any given time and you don't have to be hard on yourself. But now it is time to choose again. Choose to take wonderful, loving care of yourself and your magnificent world. Look within for guidance and for the answers to your questions. If you are willing and open, you will find what you are looking for and have been seeking. If you have been searching far and wide, stop. Be still. Listen.

I agree wholeheartedly with Erich Fromm's statement, "Our highest calling in life is precisely to take loving care of ourselves." In simply doing that, I believe we can enrich the quality of life on this planet. *You* make a difference. Our bodies are made up of trillions of cells—all of these cells constitute our person. In order to maintain perfect health, each of these cells must operate at peak performance. If we have sick or weak cells, then our healthy cells must work harder so that the body as a whole can be healthy, can work in harmony.

Our planet is like a body and we are all its individual cells. We are all waves in the same ocean. We are not separate from our fellow humans. There is no room for negative thinking, a withholding of forgiveness, bitterness toward others, or selfishness. Whenever we create an imbalance in one area of the world, there is an imbalance in the rest of the world. In other words, what happens in one area ultimately affects the rest of the world. It is *our responsibility* to this body that we call our planet to be a healthy, happy, peaceful cell that radiates only goodness, positiveness, and love. In this way we can help make our world perfect and harmonious. One person's consciousness of wellness, peace, and joy, with its outer manifestations, releases more light into human consciousness for the benefit of all.

Although the physical body and the body of humanity work along the same principles of harmony and cooperation, there is one difference. The cells of the body don't choose how they function. There is an inherent working and functioning wisdom that seems to take charge most of the time. But people do choose how they live and cooperate with one another. In other words, cooperation is not compelled. Harmony is not thrust upon us. We have a choice. And when we choose not to work together harmoniously, when we elect to stay separate and uncooperative, we experience collective illness—just as the body experiences disease when its components don't work well together. When we do work well together in cooperation, with compassion, we experience collective well-being—life as it is meant to be. This is the key to creating a world of peace and aliveness: harmonious cooperation.

The separation and division that has so long colored our thoughts and beliefs regarding our lives on this planet must now be examined and corrected. To create peace on Earth, we must stop dividing the world, the nations, the races, the religions, the sexes, the ages, the families, and the resources, and know that it's time to come together and live in harmony and love. (*Universe* literally means "one song".) Jesus, the greatest teacher who ever lived, said "Love one another." The awareness of our oneness must precede our thoughts and actions as a part of our belief system. It's your choice. You can choose to make a difference with the way you live *your* life.

In his insightful book, *The Hundredth Monkey*, Ken Keyes, Jr., tells us of a phenomenon that scientists observed when they studied the eating habits of Macaque monkeys. (This monkey research can be found in the book *A New Science of Life*, by Rupert Sheldrake.) One monkey discovered that by washing sweet potatoes before eating them, they tasted better. She taught her mother and friends until one day there were a certain number (say ninety-nine) of the monkeys who knew how to wash their sweet potatoes. The next day, when the hundredth monkey learned how to wash sweet potatoes, an amazing thing happened. The rest of the colony miraculously knew how to wash their potatoes too. Not only that, but the monkeys on *other* islands *all* started washing their potatoes. Keyes applies this "hundredth monkey" phenomenon to humanity. When more of us individually choose to make a difference with our lives—when we realize we do make a difference and start acting like it, more and more of us will hop on the bandwagon, until we reach the "millionth person" and peace spreads across the globe!

We are interconnected divine beings, working as one. When something affects the body positively, like exercise, it has a positive effect on the mind. By the same token, lack of exercise, which deteriorates the body, has a negative effect on the mind. You can't expect to experience vibrant health if you don't exercise or if you eat junk food every day. Moreover, you can exercise daily and eat the best quality food available, but if your mind and thoughts are continually negative and stressful, if you expect negative results, your health will suffer. If your life lacks a balance of activity and play, your health will suffer. What you need to do is become a master of your life, and a master in the art of living.

Here is what James Michener has to say about being a master in the art of living. "The Master in the Art of Living draws no distinction between his work and his play, his labor and his leisure, his mind and his body, his education and his recreation, his love and his religion. He hardly knows which is which. He simply pursues his vision of excellence through whatever he is doing and leaves it to others to decide whether he is working or playing, to himself he is always doing both."

When you live within nature's laws, health, joy, and peace are naturally yours, and you are a master of your life. This doesn't mean that ahead of you lies a life of boredom and sacrifice. On the contrary, good health practices can be as rewarding in the doing as they are in the results. And good health is not only an end in itself, it is the means to all other ends as well. Be true to all that you were created to be. Choose to be true to yourself—live fully and celebrate life.

At the end of the book, I have included a resource directory for those interested in finding out more about any of the people, ideas, companies, foundations, or products mentioned in the book.

Each chapter of this book is followed by questions and ideas which are designed to support you in learning more about yourself and in applying the material presented in this book to your life in a direct and personal way. Space is available for you to write your responses in the book, which will assist you in deeper study and self-discovery, and provide future reference. Don't skip over this part.

Self-Discovery Questions

1. *What does it mean to me to be healthy?*

2. *What value have I gotten from being ill in the past (for example, by being sick, someone might pay more attention to me)?*

3. *In the past, whom (or what situations) have I blamed for my failures?*

4. *People treat me in accordance with how I've taught them to treat me, that is, how I treat myself. What changes can I make in myself and my behavior that will support my newfound magnificence?*

5. *In the past I may have felt limited in what I could be or do because of what others have said. As I let go of limiting opinions and beliefs and tune in to my own inner signals, what new possibilities become exciting and available to me?*

Action Choices

1. *Following is a list of at least five things I love about myself.*

2. *Following is a list of some things I am going to change or improve about myself.*

3. *These are a few things I can do to increase my self-confidence and self-image.*

4. *Because I must take myself with me everywhere I go, I now choose to start loving myself unconditionally and consistently. In the following space I describe myself as the radiant being that I am.*

5. *I now choose to find myself more attractive than ever before. I am wonderful. I now take a few minutes to mentally picture myself as the exquisite person I am, emphasizing my many positive qualities.*

CHAPTER 2

CHOOSE TO

B E   W E L L

*Each patient carries his own doctor inside
him.*

—Albert Schweitzer

*I have learned never to underestimate the
capacity of the human mind and body to
regenerate—even when prospects seem most
wretched. The life force may be the least
understood force on earth.*

—Norman Cousins

Until recently Peter hadn't seen a physician for several years.
When his family, friends, or associates got the flu or a cold, he
would always stay healthy. This was the story he related in one of
my week-long seminars, "Wellness and Wholeness," last summer.
For Peter, all of a sudden his luck changed. A year ago he caught
a bad cold that stayed with him for a couple of weeks. Then only
a month later, Peter had a terrible sore throat that turned into a
deep, penetrating cough that lasted close to three months. Was it
coincidence that his illnesses blossomed only a few months following a brief separation from his wife, along with dissatisfaction on
the job?

Benjamin Franklin said, "Anything that hurts, instructs." When
you are feeling sick, treat it as nature's way of getting your atten-

17

tion. It's as though we all have our internal psychiatrist who tries to let us know when we need to make better choices. Quite often our sickness, in one way or another, is related to stress.

I know that I have had the experience of catching a cold when under extra stress. And I can also recall times when I have felt sure I would not get sick even though a virus was running rampant and almost everyone I knew had it. Has that ever happend to you? Perhaps you felt that you simply could not afford to get sick because of some commitment you wanted to keep. It was as if you asserted your will to keep going and your immune system cooperated.

The study of the fact that you have control over your wellness and can choose to be healthy and functioning fully is a new science that's rapidly gaining in popularity. From around the world immunologists, psychiatrists, endocrinologists, neuroscientists, microbiologists, and psychologists, who rarely step out of their own fields, are coming together to unite their fields of expertise in this new field called psychoneuroimmunology. This field deals with how your mind can affect your immune system's complex network of organs, vessels, and white blood cells. Research in this fascinating area indicates that the immune system, brain, and other vital body systems communicate with and influence one another. If your brain allows your stress level to get out of control, this can have a detrimental impact on the immune system, suppressing its ability to fight disease. In other words, if you are chronically distressed or anxious or tense, these emotions may manifest themselves as arthritis, heart disease, a kidney ailment, even cancer. On the other hand, well-managed stress can help keep your immune system healthy. That is to say, if you are happy and well-adjusted, your body will maintain its disease-fighting forces at peak capacity.

Thus by adjusting our mental outlook, we can prevent the onset of disease or lessen its impact once it strikes. This viewpoint was first reported by Soviet scientists, although they were initially ridiculed by conservative immunologists, who argued that immune responses should be observed in the test tube, with no intervention from the mind. But in speaking of the research of the past ten years, Dr. Novera Herbert Spector, a neurophysiologist at the National

Institutes of Health in Bethesda, Maryland, says, "The new research makes it clear that attitudes can matter."

I first became aware of this field when my friend Carolyn Murray, M.D., sent me a poignant article by Robert M. Mack, M.D. from the December 1984 *New England Journal of Medicine*. Entitled "Lessons from Living with Cancer," the article was an inspiration to me. Robert Mack turned 50 in 1979 and had his share of stress. He was a busy surgeon. During the previous year and a half, he and his wife divorced, his father died, one child left for college, another went to live with his ex-wife, he moved from his home to an apartment, and two family members required unexpected major surgery. In his article he describes his difficult time. He had heard, he recalls, "warnings about the stress levels in my life and the likelihood of an associated major illness. I felt helpless to alter my life...to cope differently with life's stresses. I had also once been a long-time cigarette smoker, although I had completely stopped smoking several years ago." But he had never expected to come down with cancer—an adenocarcinoma of the lung.

The cancer was detected early, and the chance for Mack's two-year survival was 50 percent. To improve his odds Mack assumed an active mental and physical role in his treatment, to complement conventional therapy. Following the advice outlined in *Getting Well Again*, by O. Carl Simonton and Stephanie Simonton (a husband-and-wife radiotherapist-psychologist team) and James Creighton, Mack pursued a "whole-person approach" to recovery from cancer.

The Simonton method calls on the patient to alter emotions, attitudes, and expectations in combating disease. Important to the process are daily exercises in relaxation and imaging and physical activity, which are intended to reduce the stresses the Simontons say play a role in disease. In Mack's case, the treatment was designed to bolster his immune system's fight against the invading cancer cells.

The Simontons state that one's wellness or illness involves not just simply the physical body, but rather the whole person, incorporating both the body and the mind. "Their theory is that patients with cancer can participate actively in the enhancement of health and the strengthening of bodily defenses," says Mack. "My coun-

selor has been instrumental in teaching me to achieve deep relaxation easily and her coaching in imagery has helped me to acquire
the valuable ability to visualize progress in my battle against cancer.
I try to achieve a state of deep relaxation at least once a day. During
those periods of calm and detachment I construct mental pictures
of what I want to happen in my battle against the cancer and in my
response to treatment. I visualize an enhancement of my immune
defenses against the cancer cells. I try to see momentarily a full
restoration of health and the absence of tumor. The desired images
do not always come readily and sometimes not at all, but those
periods of withdrawal are always restorative even when I do not
achieve the desired images."

This mental therapy uses emotions to prod certain brain chemicals into stimulating the body's defense systems against the invading disease. By the same token, the repression of emotions can
depress the body's ability to fight disease, making us sick, scientists
claim.

"If you get angry and that emotion doesn't get discharged, the
resulting hormonal products and small particles such as neurotransmitters and endorphins don't get used," says Dr. Caroline
Sperling, a clinical psychologist and director of the Cancer Counseling Institute in Bethesda, Maryland. "So they sink down, but
they don't go away. The residue remains and can become toxic in
our bodies."

The opposite, however, is also true. "When you release those
emotions effectively, you get real well-being and adrenal charging
so that the immune system stays strong and the body stays
healthy."

Following in the footsteps of the Simontons, Dr. Paul Rosch,
president of the American Institute of Stress in New York, agrees
that exciting work is going on in the field of psychoneuroimmunology, particularly in the area of visual imagery and cancer. "It has
been determined that negative emotions have a high link to certain
types of malignancies, and support for that comes from the obser-
vation that there are receptor sites on T-cell lymphocytes for certain
brain chemicals, which suggests that there is a conversation going
back and forth between the immune system and the brain."

Dr. Caroline Sperling says, "Imagery works like a computer to program into the hypothalamus the directions you want. It helps open up the parasympathetic nervous system so your body gets healthy. In other words, you're giving messages to your body, which translates them into neurotransmitters and whatever to get the immune system to work better and the hormone system to calm down a little and stop creating abnormal cells."

Some of the most promising work in the field of mental healing is being done by Dr. Candace Pert and colleagues at the National Institute of Mental Health in Bethesda, Maryland. One area of research there involves neuropeptide receptors—special brain-produced proteins that studies show have a strong effect on emotions and behavior.

"My fantasy—it's not even at the level of a hypothesis yet—is that each neuropeptide may represent a different emotion," Pert says in a *Washington Post* article.

If such were the case, it might be possible to control or prevent disease through the manipulation of these unique chemicals, researchers state.

All of the doctors who examined Dr. Caroline Sperling say she should be dead by now—the victim of breast cancer with metastasis into the abdomen. They gave her three years to live—tops. That was more than seven years ago, and she is still going strong.

Proper medical care has played an important role, and Sperling also credits sound psychological care with pulling her through the trauma: In a book in progress she discusses her experience with terminal illness.

The bottom line for patients with life threatening disease is merely this: "I am going to live no matter what that decision means in terms of changes in my life.

When patients are willing to make that kind of commitment, they are often able to mobilize their physical and emotional resources, more frequently tending to get well than could be expected from statistical probabilities alone. The quality of life is improved for all patients regardless of the outcome of their disease.

The trouble is that people often just give up at the diagnosis, but if you hang in there and learn the lessons, then it changes your life around for the better.

Hope is, I believe, the essential ingredient that energizes the body's healing efforts and maximizes its response to medical treatment.

I believe that any treatment can only support the body's own efforts at healing and I abhor the arrogance of practitioners who indicate otherwise. We do not yet know all about the mechanisms such as hormones, neurotransmitters, neuropeptides, endorphins and more by which hope and anticipation... get translated into the balances of immune activity and the interaction of biochemical processes that we call health.

Dr. Mack shared Dr. Sperling's feelings. He was determined to truly participate in his battle with cancer. He says, "I had to be willing to make decisions to alter my behavior, to become a different sort of person. I had to learn to act in ways that had not seemed feasible or permissible before. There was no guarantee that attitudinal or behavior changes on my part would alter the course of the cancer, but I became convinced that adding hope, love, and positive expectations and trying to shape a slower, more gentle life could do no harm and might be beneficial."

He started by making some changes in his lifestyle.

The first change that seemed important was to reduce the intensity of my professional life. Could I give up or at least slow down my surgical activities if it meant survival? I began taking a full day off each week. I was no longer available 24 hours a day, seven days a week. I began closing the office at four o'clock.

Then a couple years later,

I was able to make the decision to stop doing major operations, and a few months later, to stop being a primary surgeon on any operation. I still greatly enjoy assisting, and I feel valued and useful helping my long-time friend and associate, who is also a highly capable vascular surgeon.

One of the really ironic things about the human experience is that many of us have to face pain or injury or even the possibility of death in order to learn the real purpose of being and how best to live a rewarding life. My priorities, pleasures, and expectations began to change. I came to realize that I could have whatever aspirations I chose to have, in spite of the diagnosis of cancer. I believe that each of us can affect our own life and health, perhaps even our death, through our attitudes toward life and toward the treatment we are undergoing.

This whole experience of disease and survival has certainly strengthened my belief in the dependence on an Almighty power beyond my own. I have for years been agnostic in my approach to religion. However the role that I believe faith, hope, and communication with some Universal Power have in my survival and the strength I have received from the faith and prayers of those who support me have convinced me that there is an Almighty Power ill-defined in my mind but indubitably aiding me in my struggle.

Mack's attitude about life changed as a result of his life-threatening disease. He became aware of things that previously had rarely caught his attention.

I began to focus on choosing to do things every day that promote laughter, joy, and satisfaction. I decide on things like spending time alone in my garden, watching a basketball game, reading an interesting book or article, taking a slow and gentle walk at dusk with my partner, enjoying the earth and its beauty. I began to make choices to do the things that felt good to me—to allow myself the privilege of cherishing thoughts about when to plant the peas, how much manure to use, and whether there are as many primrose blossoms as I expected. I enjoy the changes season by season in the flowers, the trees, the grass, the water, and the sky. I appreciate each of these wonders. When I take the time really to look and think about them, to let them have value for me, I am not being concerned about my impending death. I enjoy all the wonderful relationships I have. I am happier than I have ever been. These are truly among the best days of my life.

His attitude about the importance of laughter is shared by Norman Cousins. Cousins has been my greatest teacher in the field of mental healing. In his excellent book *Anatomy of an Illness* he describes how he made a miraculous recovery from a long, debilitating illness. Laughter was one tool Cousins used in a conscious effort to mobilize his will to live. Long-time editor of *Saturday Review* and now a senior lecturer in medicine at UCLA, Cousins had a disease called ankalosing spondylitis. A specialist assessed his chances of recovering from this progressive and "incurable" disease as one in five hundred. Cousins felt that that would certainly be the case if he lingered in the hospital, harassed with injections and X rays and pain medications, so he checked out of the hospital and into a hotel, and proceeded, in conjunction with his doctor, to devise his own treatment plan.

His plan had three parts. First, to stop all medication, on the grounds that painkillers are potentially toxic and inhibit the body's self-healing processes. Second, he took massive amounts of vitamin C intravenously. Third, and perhaps most important, he set out to reverse the disease process by cultivating the positive emotions of love, hope, faith, laughter, and the will to live.

For laughter, Cousins turned to humor collections and old "Candid Camera" films. He noted that ten minutes of genuine belly laughter would afford him at least two hours of blissful, pain-free sleep. His unconventional regimen proved most successful, and the once-crippled patient now plays tennis and golf.

His book is a modern masterpiece on holistic health, psychoneuroimmunology, and mental healing. My favorite chapter is the one on placebos, where he intelligently explores such interesting phenomena as the placebo effect, and the effect of positive emotions on the healing process.

I remember an experience in high school where laughter came to my rescue. I was attending U. S. Grant High School in Van Nuys, California. One of my dreams was to be a cheerleader, even though I knew if I made the squad, I would be terrified being in front of an audience. I tried out and made the team a week before our first fall football game, which was to be held in the stadium at Los Angeles Valley College, across the street from the high school. For the week prior to the first game, I was so terrified that I felt sick, my muscles ached, and I had hives covering most of my body. But something happened the night before my first game that convinced me about the power of laughter, letting go, and expressing feelings in alleviating stress and improving health.

I got together with the other cheerleaders in a last-minute attempt to perfect our routines. What started out as a serious encounter turned into a joyous, hilarious adventure. We all laughed so hard we could barely stand up straight. And in between fits of laughter, we all shared our feelings of fright, low self-confidence, and excitement. After four hours of laughing and talking, even before I left the party, all my hives disappeared and I was eagerly anticipating the next day's game. By the time I went to bed that evening, my muscle aches and sick feelings brought on by the stress had vanished.

The game turned out to be lots of fun. Our school won and I learned one of the most valuable lessons of my life—the value of laughing, enjoying life, and letting go of anxiety. It sure can enhance health.

Not long ago Norman Cousins was on a local TV talk show discussing the body-mind connection. Of particular interest to me was his discussion about the body moving along the path of its expectations. For example, he talked about an experiment conducted with people about to have surgery. They were divided into two groups. The first group dreaded the surgery and did everything they could to avoid it. The second group, who had similar medical problems, regarded the surgery as a blessing and a chance to free themselves of their illness. When the surgery was over, those who had been confident and had looked forward to the surgery had a much better postoperative experience than the other group. This outcome has been repeated time and again.

Cousins also remarked about a group of cancer survivors in Santa Monica, California, who have all lived past the time predicted for them by their physicians. Why? The one thing they have in common is that they don't deny their diagnosis, but they all deny the verdict. They have a blazing determination. Their expectations are not negative and that has made the difference.

What are your thoughts about being healthy? Do you think only healthy, alive thoughts? Or do you focus on those things you dislike about your body and how you feel? Do you expect to get sick each winter or do you let go of thoughts of sickness?

I recommend some books in this area. One of my favorites is *Love, Medicine & Miracles*, by Bernie S. Siegel, M.D., which explores the common psychological characteristics of this surgeon's patients who have recovered from serious illnesses, mostly cancer. *Imagery in Healing*, by Jeanne Achtenberg, discusses how mental imagery may help patients through painful events such as childbirth as well as serious illness. One of the chapters is on the physiology and biochemistry of healing and pain relief, which, like all chapters in this book, is prodigiously referenced. *Will To Be Well*, by Neville Hodgkinson, presents in clear, straightforward language the evidence for a mind-body link in connection·with disease. Each chapter concludes with holistic, disease-specific advice that includes a mental component. *The Healer Within*, by Steven Locke, M.D., is a thorough review of the science of psychoneuroimmunology that is detailed, yet readable. Few references are given, but the book includes a lengthy appendix of organizations and other resources to turn to for further help.

Another book you may want to peruse is *Nutrition and Your Immune System*, by Carlson Wade. This book looks at your body's immune system, from defining the system and how it works to discussing diseases that are caused by a weakened immune system. Wade discusses how a strong immune system helps your body defend and repair itself, and how antibodies are your protection against illness. He also devotes sections to specific diseases: arthritis, cancer, stress, and sexually transmitted diseases. Of particular interest is the section on the "magic nutrients" that help strengthen the immune system. Finally, you may want to check out the book *You Can Heal Your Life* by Louise Hay. It beautifully shows you that all healing must first begin with self-worth and self-acceptance and honoring that part of you which is pure love.

The June 1986 issue of *National Geographic* has a superb article that not only explains in lay terms how our immune system works but is replete with incredible pictures of the immune system. The pictures presented in this feature truly describe the article's title—

"Our Immune System-The Wars Within." Written by Peter Jaret and with photographs by Lennart Nilsson, this article is an enlightening one. I was touched by the pictures of children combining fun and therapy at the M. D. Anderson Hospital in Houston, Texas. Using a video game, they zap cancer cells with the "Killer T Cell," as it has been found that visualizing enemies and protectors may positively influence the immune system. (Another excellent magazine article is *East West*, November 1986 by Kirk Johnson called *"The Mind and Immunity."*)

Many exciting studies of psychoneuroimmunology have been undertaken. In one landmark study Steven Schleifer and his colleagues at Mt. Sinai School of Medicine in New York had fifteen husbands of women with advanced breast cancer give blood samples every six to eight weeks during their wives' illnesses and for up to fourteen months after the women died. Although none of the men showed a depressed lymphocyte response while their wives were ill, their white cell response was significantly lowered as early as two weeks after their wives died and for up to fourteen months later. Schleifer believes this shows that, contrary to earlier studies, bereavement, not the experience of the spouses' illness, lowers immunity.

Prompted by his observations of the bereaved widowers, Schleifer wondered if serious depression would also be reflected in a weakened immunity. When he took blood samples from eighteen depressed patients at Mt. Sinai and the Bronx Veterans Administration Hospital, he found their lymphocytes were significantly less responsive to mitogens (substances that mimic the behavior of microorganisms by stimulating the white cells to divide) than those of healthy individuals from the general population matched for age, sex, and race.

At the University of California, San Francisco, Medical School, asthmatics who used a visualization technique to "travel through the body" to troubled cells showed improved breathing and needed less medication than those in control groups.

At the University of California, San Francisco, psychiatrists Andrew Kneier and Lydia Temoshok tested a hypothesis that heart patients and cancer patients lie at opposite ends of an anxiety profile. Electrodes were attached to the skin of subjects (twenty with heart disease, twenty with cancer, and twenty disease-free). Each subject was shown a number of unpleasant written statements designed to provoke anxiety, such as "You deserve to suffer" or "You're ugly." After seeing each, the patients were asked to mark on a scale of 0 to 10 how much the statement bothered them. The self-reports were compared with the electrical responses picked up from the skin, which were considered more accurate indicators of arousal.

What they found was that heart patients reported anxiety at a higher level than their physiological scores indicated, which is consistent with the anxious, hard-driving Type A personality that we associate with heart disease. On the other hand, cancer patients reported lower anxiety than their skin tests indicated, which the researchers concluded was an indicator of repressed emotions. Scores for the disease-free subjects fell in between.

In the same vein, researchers have looked at the emotions of those with AIDS and herpes. Lydia Temoshok, M.D., found that patients with the skin cancer melanoma who openly expressed their feelings of anger and distress regarding the disease had a lower rate of cancer-cell division and more lymphocytes than patients who withheld their feelings. Temoshok is also examining people with AIDS to determine whether their attitude affects behaviors that play a role in the prevention and treatment of the disease.

At the UCLA Medical Center, psychologist Margaret Kimeny is focusing her attention on herpes. She has found that people who have herpes and are depressed report more outbreaks of the sores than do sufferers who are not depressed. The depressed people, she also found, had lower levels of suppressor cytotoxic T cells, which help control viral infections.

But not everyone agrees that there is such a clear-cut link between the mind and health. In a ninety-page treatise published in the *Journal of Behavioral Medicine*, Dr. Bernard Fox of the National Cancer Institute reviews more than three hundred studies on cancer and the psyche. He writes that although a number of investigators had reported a link between the disease and psychological factors, many studies had failed to examine such nonpsychological variables as exposure to physical agents (such as asbestos) or chemical agents (such as cigarette smoke), the presence of medications (some of which have cancer-causing side effects), genetic predisposition, or age. These and other factors might be the real cause of the patient's cancer—or might obscure the real cause.

Similarly, in a controversial editorial in the *New England Journal of Medicine*, senior deputy editor and pathologist Marcia Angell says that the media have sold the public a bill of goods on the connection between mental state and disease. She notes that popular literature is full of "heal thyself" incantations, such as Norman Cousins's laughter-and-vitamin C remedy for disease and the Simonton program, which teaches cancer patients to imagine their healthy white blood cells gobbling up tumors. Angell fears that regimens like these may instill enormous guilt in patients who succumb to illness despite all their attempts to maintain a positive attitude.

Neurophysiologist Dr. Novera Herbert Spector agrees with Angell on one point only—patients should not be made to feel guilty about their illness. But, he says, popular conceptions that the mind influences the body are not necessarily inaccurate: "The public is sometimes ahead of the medical community." Laughter and a cheerful spirit, he says, are useful in creating a relaxed environment in the body so that the immune system can function better.

Stress and anxiety seem to affect the immune systems of animals too. In one experiment, for example, behavioral immunologist Mark Laudenslager and colleagues at the University of Denver gave mild electric shocks to twenty-four rats. Half the animals could switch off the current by turning a wheel in their enclosure, and the other half could not. The rats in the two groups were paired so that each time one rat turned the wheel it protected both itself and its helpless partner from the shock. Laudenslager found that the immune response was depressed below normal in the helpless rats but not in those that could turn off the electricity. What he has demonstrated, he believes, is that lack of control over an event, not the experience itself, is what weakens the immune system.

Other researchers agree. Jay Weiss, a psychologist at Duke University School of Medicine, has shown that animals who are allowed to control unpleasant stimuli don't develop sleep disturbances, ulcers, or changes in brain chemistry typical of stressed rats. But if the animals are confronted with situations they have no control over, they later behave passively when faced with experiences they can control. Such findings reinforce psychiatrists' suspicions that the experience or perception of helplessness is one of the most harmful factors in depression.

The following animal study was the most startling to me on how the mind can alter the immune response. In 1975 psychologist Robert Ader at the University of Rochester School of Medicine and Dentistry conditioned mice to avoid saccharin by simultaneously feeding them the sweetener and injecting them with a drug that both suppressed their immune systems and caused stomach upsets. Associating the saccharin with the stomach pains, the mice quickly learned to avoid the sweetener. In order to extinguish the taste aversion, Ader reexposed the animals to saccharin, this time without the drug, and was astonished to find that those rodents that had received the highest amounts of sweetener during their earlier conditioning died. He could only speculate that he had so successfully conditioned the rats that saccharin alone now served to weaken their immune systems enough to kill them.

If you can depress the immune system by conditioning, it stands to reason you can boost it in the same way. Novera Herbert Spector directed a team at the University of Alabama, Birmingham, that confirmed that hypothesis. The researchers injected mice with a chemical that enhances natural killer cell activity while simultaneously exposing the rodents to the odor of camphor, which has no detectable effect on the immune system. After nine sessions, mice exposed to the camphor alone showed a large increase in natural killer cell activity.

Of course, not all the evidence is in yet. Until such time, you are on your own in choosing how you will live your life and how you will take care of mental or physical challenges. But you may wish to consider that famous John Milton quotation, "The mind is its own place, and in itself can make heaven of hell, and a hell of heaven."

I know where I stand. I have an unshakable belief in the power
of will, faith, and hope to help us in handling all types of problems.
For more than a decade now, I've done counseling individually and
in groups; some of my clients have major illnesses. My approach
includes seeing the positive side of all circumstances, choosing to
be in charge and to not feel hopeless, and, of course, lots of laughter. Rather than sitting indoors, many of my sessions are conducted
outside in nature, walking by the beach, hiking in the mountains,
or sitting by a stream. Being in a peaceful, beautiful environment
is the thing my participants say they like the best. It helps them to
feel peaceful inside, to let go of negative emotions, and to open themselves up to the spirit of life.

No sickness can be treated on the physical level alone. The whole
person must be treated. As someone once said, "It's not the disease
that is important, but the person who has the disease." And no matter
what the treatment, the patient's faith, hope, and will to live can
make or break any remedy. "We doctors do nothing. We only help
and encourage the doctor within," Albert Schweitzer once said.

There are so many things you can do to keep your immune system in tune. Many of these will be discussed in great detail in the
rest of this book. Briefly, however, pay close attention to the following guidelines.

Eat wholesome foods, exercise regularly, drink plenty of water,
and avoid cigarettes, alcohol, caffeine, and other drugs that may interfere with your immune functioning.

Take some time out each day to relax and be still. Relaxation exercises are invaluable for eliminating stress. They allow you to become
deeply relaxed in mind and body. Meditation is another excellent
way to relax. Other ways to relax are through yoga or relaxation tapes.
(All of my audiocassettes, with the exception of the nutrition tape
#3, have a different relaxation guided imagery exercise.) Don't kid
yourself: a few drinks or a weekly dip in a hot tub are just not the
same as bringing about thorough relaxation by using your own mind
and will.

Surround yourself with family and friends who will be with you
and support you without judgment or criticism. In my life I

have learned how important this is for self-acceptance and self-esteem. As I am embraced by loving and caring friends, I blossom, and am even more willing to give back the same. The positive energy exchange between friends who have an unconditional love for each other is truly calming and nurturing. Dr. Mack expresses these sentiments aptly in his article.

> I have received tremendous positive energy and support from a variety of people who have expressed concern and caring. I have felt warmed and strengthened as the people around me have reached out and let me know that they are grateful for my presence. Somehow, being valued by others enhances my worth. My sense of control is heightened. The people who have said that I am important to them have nourished the me that I would like to be and am intent on becoming. I have learned to love and to allow myself to be loved by many people in my life and to allow closeness, caring, and touching from many, many people. It has been said that love cures people, both those who give it and those who receive it. Certainly, both giving and receiving love are wonderfully rewarding.

And about his counselor, who helped him through his challenge, he said,

> She is, without question, a major factor in my still being alive, and well, and functioning. The first session we had was an exhilirating experience. I had always been somewhat skeptical about counselors, but in this instance I felt heard, understood, and appreciated. There was a lot to learn and to begin to accept. I think that each person who has cancer or any life-threatening illness needs to find a sensitive, safe, and nonjudgmental listener—a counselor of some sort who can guide the patient through the tough spots. The counselor must be sensitive and perceptive, able to suggest available choices as well as to clarify concerns and anxieties. . . . I needed help and was fortunate that my counselor had the necessary knowledge and skills and was a person with whom I could relate without concern about being judged or rejected.

Watch your thoughts and stop them from pointless wandering. Always keep your mind and thoughts attuned to the positive side of every situation. Release every negative thought from your mind. I began doing this years ago by starting with just one hour. During that time I worked on entertaining only healthy, uplifting, self-supporting thoughts. About every five minutes or so a negative thought would pop up, and I noticed how negativity breeds negativity. I can't say it's easy to be positive all the time, but I started with one hour, and then gradually worked up to one day, and then to one week, and so on. What I discovered was that much of my thinking was habitual. Today I am very positive and in control of most of my thought process rather than letting my thoughts control me. That's not to say that every once in awhile a negative idea doesn't pop in, but when it does, I recognize it quickly and send it on its way. I also have a few friends that I have asked to help me be positive and when I slip, they gently remind me what I've done.

Watch out for stress associated with prolonged feelings of anger, depression, helplessness, or hopelessness. Negative emotions trigger the release of substances that can suppress immune functioning. If a contract falls through or someone in your family is upset about something you did, pay attention to solving the problem in a way that lets you clear up your negative feelings as thoroughly and quickly as possible. One of the greatest gifts you can give another human being is to encourage that person to express feelings. It's a gift of health for both of you. I know that sometimes it can be difficult, and it does take practice. But stick with it. Your life may depend on it.

Be aware that your immune system can take a nosedive after a traumatic event or after many seemingly inconsequential changes. Take particularly good care of yourself during the grieving period following any loss, whether it is the resignation of a talented employee, a divorce, or the death of a friend or family member.

Maintain a sense of organization and control over your personal life and work life. Research suggests that lack of control over important life circumstances is linked to immune system dysfunction. This does not mean it is necessary to control others, just your own perceptions and feelings.

Any person you have ever held a grudge against, anyone you resent, anyone you feel has hurt you in any way, forgive that individual. This is probably the biggest step you can take toward the enhancement of your immune system. Begin with forgiving yourself. There are many excellent exercises for practicing forgiveness of yourself and others in the wonderful books *Practical Spirituality*, by John R. Price, and *Living in the Light*, by Shakti Gawain.

Develop a sense of humor and a healthy degree of emotional detachment and hearty laughter. This can stimulate the immune system and make your days be filled with joy and happiness.

Finally, give three or more hugs every day. My mom taught me the importance of hugging many years ago. (Leo Buscaglia, professor of education at the University of Southern California, also known as the love guru, cites scientific studies showing that men who hug and kiss their wives before they go to work and when they return home live longer and have less illness than those who are not as demonstrative. "C'mon guys. If this is all it is, let's wake up," Buscaglia urges.) Further, find ways that you can serve your fellow human beings and be as caring, kind, and loving as you can. Dr. Mack found this to be a special part of his program.

In the fall of 1985, Mack, after two years without evidence of progression of cancer, discovered some other complications with his blood flow. Yet, for Mack, attitude continued to play a key role in his fight against the odds. "I think my attitudes have continued to be positive. I feel I have some worth left, and I want to be able to expend it as well as I can and as long as I can. I think with having a positive attitude about living and contributing, even if I can't be a surgeon any longer—and I'm not—I can pass on some knowledge, some caring, some loving and some hugging to people and help them with their attitudes."

On December 20, 1985, Robert Mack died from complications of his illness. He died in his sleep while the imagery tapes he used to relax played.

Self-Discovery Questions

1. *Here are many reasons why I deserve to be optimally healthy and fully functioning.*

2. *What am I feeling angry about? This is how I'll let the anger go.*

3. *What am I feeling upset about? This will help me let the feeling go.*

4. *What am I feeling depressed and hopeless about? I'll release it by doing this.*

5. *What am I feeling happy and joyful about?*

6. *In the past I have chosen to feel anxious about the following things. I now choose to let this anxiety go.*

7. *When can I set aside time each day to be by myself and to relax?*

8. *I can ask the following people to help me to be positive.*

9. *Identify times of particular stress in your past and see if there was a correlation with your health.*

Action Choices

1. *Sit quietly with your eyes closed for the next few minutes, envision yourself as a peaceful, relaxed, confident, and happy person. Describe how that looked and felt.*

2. *Every night before you go to sleep, sit quietly and forgive yourself and others that you feel have hurt you in any way. List those people that need your immediate attention.*

3. *Take one person with whom you have not been feeling in harmony. Close your eyes and see both of you sitting facing each other in a circle of white light. Now lovingly share your feelings with that person and resolve any conflict. Finish with seeing your hearts connect and loving each other unconditionally.*

4. *If you need to forgive a person who has died, sit down and write that individual a letter. Pour out all your feelings and finish it with offering forgiveness and love.*

5. *If you know someone who's experiencing lots of stress, anxiety, depression, hopelessness, or helplessness, contact that person as soon as possible. Encourage him or her to express feelings to you as you listen without judging, criticizing, or offering advice. Sometimes all we need is someone who cares and will take the time to listen and be our friend. List here who you'll be contacting.*

6. *From this day forward, I will give* _____ *hugs each day.*

7. *I now know that the better I handle stress, the healthier and happier I'll be. Here are some ways I've handled stress in the past. Here are the ways I now choose to deal with stress that support my immune system and well-being.*

CHAPTER 3

CHOOSE

WHAT YOU THINK, SAY, AND IMAGINE

I am responsible for what I see.
I choose the feelings.
I experience, and I decide
Upon the goal I would achieve.
And everything that seems
To happen to me I ask for
And receive as I have asked.
                    —*A Course in Miracles*

Man is made or unmade by himself. By the
right choice he ascends. As a being of power,
intelligence, and love, and lord of his own
thoughts, he holds the key to every situation.
                    —*James Allen, As A Man Thinketh*

Positive thinking became almost synonymous with success in the 1970s. In its early use in organizations such as Dale Carnegie's success courses, positive thinking meant using willpower and concious, positive thoughts to achieve goals. "What you can conceive and believe, you can achieve," is a popular positive thinking slogan.

It's a curious thing to me that no one ever taught me how to use my mind in school. I was taught mathematics, history, science, social studies, and English, but no course was offered on the science of mind so that I could learn more effectively. If I had my way, I would require all students, each year of their education, to take a class I'd call mind power. This would be the science of mind and would cover a variety of topics, including mind strength and clarity—how to be alert yet relaxed. A special section would be devoted to attention and how it affects all areas of our lives. Finally, students would be shown how to choose effective, positive thoughts—to be in control of thinking at all times, instead of allowing thoughts to be in control.

Review your thoughts through the day. Do you generally think positive or negative thoughts? Do you think that you have many thoughts? Do you think that you are in control of your thoughts? Many of us are not even aware of how much we think and how negative our thoughts are. When you wake up, are you excited about the new day? Or do your thoughts center around the discordant alarm, no time for breakfast, too much traffic on the way to work, and unhappiness with your job? The thought processes go on and on during the day. If you believe that positive thinking doesn't really matter because "How many thoughts can a person actually have during a day, anyway?"—well, give it another thought!

According to the National Science Foundation, you think thousands of thoughts every day—in fact, about 1000 an hour. When you are writing you think 2500 thoughts in about 1½ hours. The ordinary human being thinks about 12,000 thoughts a day. A deeper thinker, according to this report, puts forth about 50,000 thoughts. So imagine that 50 percent of the time you are positive in your thinking. For many of you that still means 25,000 negative thoughts you might be programming every day and, thus, the reality you are creating with your thought.

A man is what he thinks about all day long.

—Emerson

That's right. What we believe to be true and what we think about consistently—our mental atmosphere—is mirrored back to us in our surroundings. This is not merely my theory but is supported by scientists, psychologists, psychiatrists, hypnotherapists, metaphysicians, and others in the healing profession.

Inevitably, your beliefs and thoughts create your reality. Let's look at an all-too-common example of how this concept works: weight control. Let's assume that you've always had difficulty controlling your weight. You've tried all kinds of diets and they've never worked, so you have negative beliefs about diets. You've tried to limit the amount of food you eat without much success, so you don't have much faith in your self-control. And you get on the scale every morning and the figures on the scales usually serve to reinforce your view of yourself as overweight. It really is a vicious cycle. In order to better understand why you keep repeating the same patterns, let me explain a bit about the way your mind works.

Brain researchers see the mind as composed of two primary parts: the conscious mind and the subconscious mind. A window to the world, your conscious mind runs your daily waking activities, such as making decisions, relating to others, and so on. Your subconscious mind, however, carries memories of all your experiences. It is the storage center for all the information your conscious mind sends it, based on your daily experiences. Your subconscious mind is a computer that is fed the data of your every thought and experience.

Relating this to the example of weight control: if you get up every morning and worry about what clothes will fit, if you dread getting on your scale, if you dislike being seen in public, if you think about going on a diet but doubt that it will work, *you are programming your subconscious computer in a negative way.*

So you have some excess pounds on you. Rather than getting down on yourself, simply own the fact that you've deposited some extra fat on your body. You don't have to continue repeating the past. You can choose to manifest a different result—being trim and fit. Create new beliefs, thoughts, visualizations, and actions. You can reprogram yourself to create what you desire and deserve.

Your mind creates reality according to its programming. If you think of yourself as fat, as having little self-control, as being unable to change, you will see those beliefs reflected in your life.

The same is true for every other area of your life. Your beliefs and thoughts about yourself, your relationships with others, your money, your material possessions, and so on, will be faithfully recreated in your life. Now you may be reading this and thinking, "That isn't true for me. I know that I really want to lose weight and tone up my body (or make more money or get involved in a relationship) but I'm not experiencing that in my life." To that I would say that there is a difference between wanting something on a conscious level and wanting it on a subconscious level.

Our conscious mind and our subconscious mind are often in conflict. Consciously you may want something, yet subconsciously you create mediocrity or failure. That's why positive thinking as it is commonly perceived doesn't work. It doesn't do much good to force yourself to think positive thoughts on a conscious level while your subconscious still harbors many negative beliefs. What you need to do in order to break the vicious cycle of negative beliefs that is creating a negative reality is to reprogram your subconscious mind through methods we will examine in a moment. In addition, you must make some behavior changes on a conscious level that will contribute to new beliefs.

In other words, you must be what you desire. To be it, you must first capture the feeling of whatever it is you desire, whether it's being happy, or loving, or prosperous, or trim. Then you'll start acting that way and finally become it. The essential key in the process is capturing the feeling, because when you do that you've captured the ability to internalize it. Then it's only a matter of time.

If you see your world only according to what surrounds you right now, you are judging by appearances and limiting what you are going to have. Instead of thinking, "I'll believe it when I see it," think "I'll see it when I believe it." Trust in the Universe, the power within, regardless of appearances. Ernest Holmes once said, "Trust in the invisible, for it's the sole cause of that which is visible."

As we change our consciousness, we change our lives. Because thoughts create form, the very thing you believe becomes reality for you because you believe in it. Richard Bach, in *Jonathan Livingston Seagull*, said, "Don't you believe what your eyes are telling you. All they show is limitation. Look with your understanding, find out what you already know and you'll see the way to fly."

> We need only in cold blood act as if the thing in question were real and it will become infallibly real by growing in such a connection with our life that it will become real.
>
> —William James

William James, founder of one of the first psychological laboratories in this country, said that belief can be embodied in consciousness through "the path of emotions" and "the path of will." Regarding the emotions, he wrote that the idea must be one that excites our interest. The interest will then stimulate the emotions, particularly feelings of love, and when the feeling reaches the stage of passion it will then be recorded as a belief in the mind.

Regarding "the path of will," he wrote:

> Gradually our will can lead us to the same results by a very simple method. We need only *act* as if the thing in question was real, and keep acting as if it were real, and it will infallibly end by growing into such a connection with our life that it will become real. It will become so knit with habit and emotion that our interests in it will be those which characterize belief.

He also said:

> If you only care enough for a result, you will almost certainly attain it. If you wish to be rich, you will be rich. If you wish to be learned, you will be learned. If you wish to be good, you will be good. Only you must really wish these things and wish them exclusively and not wish at the same time 100 other incompatible things as strongly.

So first, you must say what it is you desire, and you must be specific. You must put in mind that which you choose to bring into your life. You must direct the power within to create what you want. The creative principle works according to the seeds that you plant. Therefore it's imperative that you plant the seeds that you desire to grow. When you plant seeds that you don't want to grow, it's out of a lack of understanding. If you plant love you get back love. If you plant scarcity, you get back scarcity. So, say what you want, be specific, and act "as if," that is, act as if what you want were already true.

It's important to understand the role of feelings in being the person you want to become. Your feelings are the power that creates. Just to simply visualize something without deep, passionate feeling will do little good. From the extensive research I have done in the field of manifestation, I have come to appreciate the role of feelings. One source described feelings as an electromagnetic force field that is so strong it sends up a vibration that pulls like vibrations to itself. It is a magnet for similar energy particles. The result: more of those situations that produced the feeling to begin with. For example, human behavior specialists know that success begets success and failure begets failure. After interviewing many highly intelligent, successful people with diverse backgrounds and vast experience, the conclusion I came to was that how you feel about things can be a determining factor in the way your life works out. And any feeling we want we can have by simply being it. It's this powerful force of feeling that acts as the generator to bring into creation that which we desire. Negative feelings will bring negative results. Positive feelings will bring positive results.

As I counsel around the country, I often hear statements such as this: "I continually affirm, visualize, meditate, and believe in my highest good, but I rarely see results." Most of the time it's because the receiving channels have not been opened. This can be done by practicing forgiveness toward ourselves and others and by releasing all fear, anger, and guilt. (More about these in Chapter 7.)

Let's now take a look at some external, conscious changes you can make. For example, if you feel that your beliefs about money are creating negative results in your life, examine the behaviors that support those negative beliefs. Maybe you are frugal in your grocery shopping; you always buy the cheapest of every brand and skip the luxuries. Although that frugality might be wise in light of your current financial situation, you should be aware that it also tends to reinforce your belief that you have very little money. One way to attack this belief would be to substitute a new behavior for an old one. In other words, the next time you're in a grocery store, allow yourself to indulge in a little luxury. And while you're doing it, imagine that this is your present reality.

If your problem is loneliness, make it a point to smile at one stranger every day, just as if you had plenty of friends and an abundance of love to share.

If you are overweight, buy yourself something appealing that you would normally have denied yourself because of your present weight.

The more time you spend acting "as if" and imagining yourself as already having achieved a goal, the more likely you will be able to achieve the goal. Psychiatrist David Viscott once said, "Happiness is the purposeful movement toward achieving meaningful goals." Aliveness comes from both moving toward your goals and achieving them.

You must also give away the very thing you desire. This is the law of circulation. What you give out, you get back multiplied. If you desire increased prosperity in your life, share what you do have with others. Don't hoard it, because that would be a manifestation of a fear that there might not be enough.

The other day, after writing my prosperity affirmations and goals on cards, I went to the grocery store. While waiting in the checkout line, I suddenly called out to the harried mother in front of me, "I'll pay for those." Well, needless to say, she was astonished. Quite honestly, so was I. The words seemed to have just popped out of my mouth. I paid her bill and I felt terrific. It is said, "To give is to receive," and it surely rang true for me that day in the market. The pleasure I received made me feel rich inside. But that is not the end of the story.

Later that same day I ran into a person whom I had counseled several months before. At that time she had been unable to pay, and so I just let it go. But that day she wrote me a check.

To act "as if" takes courage and trust, and I know it's hard to start giving when you don't think you have enough. I realize that some of you reading this want to get out there and participate and have fun, but you are scared. But you must go out into the world as if you had the courage—and then you'll find that the courage you wanted is already there. Do the thing and the power is yours. But it begins with a risk. If you don't risk you don't receive. That's how you generate the power.

Another way to move toward the achievement of our goals is through reprogramming our subconscious mind. There are many methods available: creative visualization, affirmations, meditation, hypnosis, and biofeedback techniques are just a few. The idea is to alter your state of consciousness so you can temporarily set aside the conscious mind and focus your concentration specifically on your subconscious. Suggestions given to your subconscious while in an altered state of consciousness, whether they are images or affirmations, will be at least 20 times as effective as suggestions given in a normal state of consciousness, according to brain researchers and behavioral psychologists.

Although altering your state of consciousness may sound difficult, it's really easy. In fact, you change your state of consciousness at least twice a day without realizing it: when you wake up in the morning and when you fall asleep at night. That's because you pass through different states of consciousness, or brain wave levels, as you pass into and out of sleep. According to brain researchers, four brain wave levels characterize your state of consciousness. Beta is waking consciousness. As your body becomes relaxed you move into alpha, a state of consciousness in which you are still fully aware of your environment but are probably untroubled by it. Still closer to sleep is theta. While in theta you may still maintain some conscious awareness of your environment, but your mind will be totally concentrating on the relaxed feeling in your body. Delta is the sleeping state. While in delta you are completely unconscious and have no sense of your surroundings.

For reprogramming purposes you need only be concerned with the alpha and theta levels of your mind. This is where you can speak directly to your subconscious while still maintaining conscious control of the programming you are supplying.

Before we go any further into actual techniques you can use to reprogram your subconscious and thus transform your life, I want to emphasize the importance of recognizing how your beliefs create your reality. All that you have ever dreamed, desired, or thought is what you have at this very moment. If things aren't just the way you would like them to be and you desire some changes in your life, first you must change your beliefs, thoughts, and the words you speak (as I touched on in Chapter 2).

> The greatest force in the human body is the natural drive of the body to heal itself—but that force is not independent of the belief system, which can translate expectations into physiological change. Nothing is more wonderous about the fifteen billion neurons in the human brain than their ability to convert thoughts, hopes, ideas and attitudes into chemical substances. Everything begins, therefore, with belief. What we believe is the most powerful option of all.
>
> —Norman Cousins

Many people feel that their deepest beliefs and feelings are forever a mystery to them. They feel they don't understand the real reasons behind their actions, and as a result they feel powerless to change their actions. *You have the power and ability to recognize and change the beliefs you have about yourself.* Although your beliefs may seem mysterious and complicated on a conscious level, on a subconscious level they are usually simple. *Your beliefs about yourself are based entirely on your past experiences.* All of your experiences program your subconscious, and the result is the person you are today.

That is not to say that all you will ever be is the sum of your experiences. Unless you take conscious control and choose the kind of programming you are feeding into your subconscious computer, however, you are destined to repeat your past experiences. Have you ever noticed that your life experiences are all very similar—it's just the people who keep changing?

The subconscious is programmed; it doesn't reason. When you understand this concept and integrate this knowledge into your life, you will be able to create a healthier, happier life than you ever imagined possible. The subconscious works to create reality according to the programming it has been fed. Although this is normally accomplished by thoughts and through your life experiences, brain researchers have found that *the subconscious is incapable of telling the difference between reality and fantasy, between the real experience and the imagined experience.*

The following study demonstrates this. Test subjects were placed in a room and wired to an EEG machine in order to record brain wave patterns under specific conditions. In this experiment someone ran into the room and fired a toy gun. Someone else did a dance, a dog barked, a color was projected, and many other test situations were enacted. As the subjects were exposed to each situation, it caused their brain waves to form patterns on the instrument recording paper. With each situation, a mark was noted on the recording paper corresponding to the activity that transpired to create each pattern.

Following this part of the test, the subjects were asked to sit and concentrate upon the situations described by the researchers. As an example: "I now want you to imagine someone running into the room and firing a gun. Hear it, see it, and imagine it happening right in front of you." At the same time the subject was imagining each act, the brain waves were once again being recorded. The results of the tests showed that the exact same patterns of brain wave activity were created when someone came into the room and did a dance, or the gun was shot, or the dog barked as when the subjects imagined these events. *The computer part of the brain was incapable of telling the real from the imagined.*

And then there are the numerous classic studies in which a person in a hypnotic trance is touched by an object such as a piece of ice, that is represented as a piece of hot metal. Almost invariably, a blister will develop at the point of contact. What this demonstrates is that it is not reality that counts, but belief—the direct, unquestioned communication to your nervous system. The brain does what it is told.

At the University of Chicago a study was done of visualization and sports ability. Subjects were divided into three groups and took part in an experiment based upon basketball. At the beginning all the participants were tested as to their individual basket-shooting ability and the results were recorded. Then group one was told, "You are each to practice shooting baskets for twenty minutes a day for twenty days." Group two was told, "Don't play any basketball for twenty days. In fact, just forget about basketball for the entire time." Group three was told, "You are to spend twenty minutes a day imagining you are *successfully* shooting baskets. Do this every day for twenty days. See every detail of your accomplishments in your mind." At the conclusion, the three groups were tested again. Group two members, who hadn't played basketball for twenty days, showed no improvement. Group one members, who had been practicing twenty minutes a day for twenty days, showed a 24 percent improvement in their basket-shooting ability. Group three members who had only *imagined* that they were successfully shooting baskets for twenty minutes a day, showed a 23 percent improvement in their actual basket-shooting ability—only one percentage point less than the group that had actually been practicing!

So taking time each day to visualize your goals can have a profound effect on your life. As George Bernard Shaw said, "Imagination is the beginning of creation. You imagine what you desire, you will what you imagine; and at last you create what you will."

Let's talk about the power of creative visualization and affirmation, how to use them, and how to alter your state of consciousness to make your programming more effective.

Albert Einstein said that he conceived of the theory of relativity by visualizing "what it must look like to be riding on the end of a light beam."

Henry David Thoreau once said, "If one advances confidently in the direction of his dreams, and endeavors to live the life which he has imagined, he will meet with success unexpected in common hours."

I love that. It always works, but it takes getting out there and advancing confidently in the direction of your dreams. What are your dreams? What is your vision? What do you expect to achieve in life? An important part of the process is expectation. Always expect to achieve your highest good, the best life has to offer, and live so that the best may become a part of your experience.

This moment, and always, choose consciously to take your attention off those things that you don't want in your life, and think about and visualize what you do want. As so simply, yet profoundly said by Richard Bach in *Illusions*, "What you can visualize, you can actualize." In addition, you must have faith. If you have faith in yourself, you have faith in everything. And yes, faith means sometimes having to believe in things that common sense doesn't seem to support. Faith also means living beyond what you can see with your eyes. Don't judge by appearances.

Keep close watch over your attention. It's a most precious faculty. Whatever we place our attention on is encouraged to flourish. Brain specialist Dr. Wilder Penfield said that if he had his life to live over again he would devote it to the study of human attention. Your attention is the intentional channeling of awareness, and one of the best ways I have found to prevent my attention from running wild and to keep it under my control is through a regular program of meditation—which is discussed in the last chapter.

Never allow anyone or anything to cause you to doubt your power and ability to live your vision—to manifest your goals and dreams. Decide what you want to create. Get clear on that first; there's power in clarity. Next, set some goals for yourself. There are many excellent books on goal-setting. One I recommend is *The Potential Is Within You*, by Roy Eugene Davis. I have an audiocassette on this topic called *How To Achieve Any Goal* (see resource directory). Goals are an important part of living your vision, and goals give you something constructive to think about. So many of us spend our waking hours thinking about all the negative elements around us or about how others should change to meet our expectations. Goals give our thoughts positive direction and purpose. When we know what we want and where we are headed, we don't spend our time thinking about what we don't want or don't have. Remember, what we think about consistently, we get.

This was never more apparent or real to me than it was on a ski trip I took to Sun Valley, Idaho, several years ago. Part of the UCLA Ski Club's ski package involved a flight to a city in Idaho where we later would catch a bus for the long ride to Sun Valley. I bought my ticket early and looked forward to the trip for weeks. On the day of departure my mom dropped me off at the airport, I checked in, got my seat assignment, and then boarded the plane. I was puzzled at not seeing any of my friends, who were part of this trip, on the flight. I figured they must all be sitting toward the back.

Then I became concerned when I couldn't find any of my friends at the baggage claim area. Bewildered and confused, I headed for the outdoor curb where, according to my ski information packet, the buses would be waiting. No friends or buses anywhere! I called the bus company to find out why the buses were late. Somewhat amused, the person on the other end of the line informed me, "The buses will be there tomorrow." Tomorrow! In light of the fact that I am an organized, efficient, and accountable person, you can imagine my astonishment.

How was it that I marked the wrong day on my calendar, talked with my friends about our upcoming ski trip without discovering the erroneous date, and encountered no problems at the airport when the ticket I offered had the following day's date on it?

Well, as is my style, I decided to make the best of it. I made reservations at a nearby hotel with a sauna, jacuzzi, and a salad bar. After the taxi dropped me off, I called my mom back home and we had a good laugh about my oversight. Bundling up in my sweats and ski hat, I went out for a jog in the freshly fallen snow.

After awhile I came across an inviting health food store. It had a small restaurant and I decided to get some soup. As I waited for the waitress to take my order, I became aware of an elderly man sitting a few tables away. He was staring at me with a weird expression on his face. I felt uncomfortable. Then rather quickly, his stare turned from inquisitiveness to a look of shock. I then noticed his wife asking him if he was okay. Pointing to me, he continued to stare as his wife turned in my direction.

Apprehensively, the man came to my table. Then, with difficulty in forming his words, he asked, "Are you Susan Smith Jones?" Well, I couldn't believe that someone had recognized me; I was wearing three layers of clothes and a hat. When I answered, he and his wife gasped.

It turned out that one week before, this man, sitting in the very same health food store, had read an article I had written about creative visualization. I wrote about how, through visualization, you can create any reality you choose. After reading this article, which included a picture of me, the man said to his wife how much he would like to meet and talk with me. His wife skeptically suggested that he visualize meeting me—which is exactly what he had been doing the week before we met.

One thing is certain—neither of them will ever question the validity and power of creative visualization. Nor will I. We talked for a few hours, shared many stories, and they drove me back to my hotel.

I've come to realize, from this circumstance as well as countless others, that there's an unfathomable, yet recognizable, divine order to this universe. It's ever present and always working in alignment with what we need for our highest good and spiritual unfoldment and growth.

I've learned not to analyze or question it anymore. I continue to live in awe at the magnificent adventure life continually is. I'm convinced that it's extremely important to always imagine and think about what you want in life, while at the same time letting go of thoughts of what you don't want. Let your imagination work for you and not against you. Make friends with your thoughts. Know that you are exactly where you need to be in life and, at any moment, you can choose to experience something else simply by taking responsibility and consciously choosing to think differently. This reminds me of the fantastic line by writer Nikos Kazantzakis: "You have your paintbrush and colors. Paint paradise, and in you go."

Now remember, when you use creative visualization, see your desire as an already accomplished fact. Dwell in perfect confidence, peace, and certainty, never looking for results, never wondering or becoming anxious or hurried. Above all, don't worry. Worry brings fear and fear is crippling. Really, the only thing that could be cause for worry is fearing you'll have to do it all by yourself. Know that there is a power greater than yourself within you, orchestrating your every encounter and always guiding you in the right direction. So let go of those troubling thoughts. It was Mark Twain who said, "I'm an old man and have had many troubles, most of which never happened."

If, for example, you want to lose weight and you are clear on this goal, here's what you might do. Create a mental movie (visualization) in which you see yourself walking into a clothing store and trying on a dress or suit two sizes smaller than the size you are now wearing. Imagine yourself looking in the mirror, and then experience delight when it fits. Then imagine that a sales clerk comments on how well you wear your clothes. When you take the outfit home, imagine your mate or a friend being pleased and surprised by how much weight you've lost. Then in another mental movie you might imagine yourself getting on the scale in the morning and seeing that you've achieved your desired weight. Whatever mental movies you create, keep them fresh and exciting to you. Emotion and feeling have more power in your subconscious than reasoning.

When you have completed the mental movie, create some affirmations that you can repeat to support your goal. An affirmation for a weight loss goal might be: "Every day in every way I am becoming more slender and fit."

There is power in what you say. Although it is sometimes difficult to control your thoughts, you can always control your words. Always affirm what you want in life. Words can be a blessing or a curse. Be aware of everything you say. Each word is just like a rock that we throw into a lake—the ripples fan out and spread across a large area. Every word we speak is an act of creating, just like our thoughts. There is an unwritten law that we attract to ourselves the equivalent of that which we express by our thoughts and words. That means that every time we bless or praise something we actually bring a blessing to ourselves. The opposite is also true.

Now I am not saying that all you have to do is put different pictures in your head and say a few positive words and immediately your life will turn around. I am saying that *in order to change, you must start with your images, thoughts and words.* They will then get stored in your subconscious as reality. Then you will start acting on that new reality. I use visualization for everything from healing relationships to increasing my fitness level.

Right now, take a moment and look back over your life and see how you have attracted either happiness or disaster through your words. Keep in mind that the subconscious has no sense of humor. People joke destructively about themselves, and the subconscious takes it seriously. The mental picture you make while speaking impresses the subconscious and works itself out on the external level. A person who knows the power of the word becomes careful with conversation.

After setting goals in an important area of your life, write some affirmations supporting these goals. I have provided a few sample affirmations at the end of this chapter. To affirm is to declare positively or firmly, to maintain to be true. In other words, an affirmation is a strong, positive statement that something is already so. It is a way of making firm that which you are desiring and visualizing. By using affirmations you can weed out the limiting and false beliefs you have about yourself and program those goals you wish to achieve. Don't underestimate the power of using affirmations. It is an effective technique, one that can positively affect your attitude, thoughts, and expression, thereby transforming the quality of your life in a short time.

There are a few points to keep in mind when composing your affirmations. Make sure the affirmations are in the present tense, rather than the future. Remember, the subconscious has no reasoning power and doesn't understand abstract concepts, such as the future. So rather than affirming, "I will weigh (your goal) pounds by the end of the month and my body will be firm, strong, and well-defined," say something like this: "I weigh (your goal) pounds easily and effortlessly and my body is strong, firm, and well-defined." It doesn't matter how far away from your ideal weight you are right now. This practice acknowledges that everything always begins on a mental plane and then manifests itself on the physical plane.

Next, make sure your affirmations are phrased in the positive. In other words, don't say, "I no longer feel tired or lack self-esteem." If you phrase your affirmation in this way, your subconscious may hear only the negative words. Instead, affirm, "I always have an abundance of energy and have high self-esteem."

Make up affirmations that truly have meaning for you—words that you can feel deep in your heart, affirmations that elicit emotion. It's not just a matter of perfunctorily reciting these words; you must feel them, be moved by them.

These affirmations can be used alone or with visualizations. For the most powerful result, use your affirmations often. Say them quietly to yourself. Say them out loud. Make a recording of your affirmations and play them several times each week. (One of the seven audiocassettes from my *Celebrate Life!* program, "Affirm a Beautiful Life," contains numerous affirmations focusing on being healthy and living fully; it includes background music.) I also recommend that you write your affirmations. You can write them individually on three-by-five-inch index cards and place them around your home and office. Also, take each affirmation and write it twenty-one times on a piece of paper, saying it as you write.

You can even work on your affirmations with others. Sit with your partner and have your partner say your affirmation to you, using your name, such as, "John, your body is trim, fit, and strong, and you look so good." To that you will reply, "Yes, I know."

As you become more familiar with using affirmations, begin to include them in your daily conversations. Make strong positive statements about yourself, situations, and people that you want to see in a more positive way. Make an agreement with a friend to support each other in choosing only positive words, and call each other on negative words. You will discover that speaking positively will become a natural way of life for you. Your reality is simply a manifestation of your thoughts and the words you speak (along with your beliefs). So choose them carefully.

How do you get the most out of your visualizatons and affirmations? Of course you should use your affirmations throughout the day along with visualizing your goals in their successful state. But for this programming to be dramatically effective, to really take hold, to bring results more quickly, set aside at least fifteen minutes each day so you can purposely alter your state of consciousness.

"Imagination is more important than knowledge."
                                                        —Albert Einstein

One of the ways you can alter your state of consciousness is quite simple. Find a place where you can be alone and undisturbed. Sit comfortably with your back straight. You can also lie down, as long as you don't fall asleep. Then breathe slowly and deeply for a few moments. As you continue to breathe slowly and deeply, imagine a wave of relaxation entering your feet. With your eyes now closed, imagine this wave slowly and progressively moving up through every part of your body, totally relaxing each body part. After you have touched every part of your body with this relaxing wave, start to vividly visualize your goal or goals. Before finishing, say the affirmations that support the reality you want to create. The entire process might take fifteen to thirty minutes. As you return to your regular state of consciousness, let go of your mental movie and bring your thoughts back to your environment. Remind yourself that you have the power and ability to create the reality you desire. You really do!

Your mind is a powerful tool for creating positive change, but it isn't always your friend. As most of you who have ever set out on a new exercise program know, your mind is often a less than willing participant.

Perhaps you've taken up jogging and made an agreement with yourself that you're going to get out there at least every other day. For the first week you have a lot of motivation, but by the second week priorities usually begin to shift. It seems that something always comes up that is more important than jogging. Perhaps you need to be in the office early in the morning and can't take time for a morning run. Or your children might begin complaining about not receiving your undivided attention. Or maybe you just stayed out too late and an extra hour's sleep seems more inviting than ten laps around the track. Whatever circumstances you create—and they always seem legitimate at the time—be aware that your mind is doing a number on you. Your mind is creating excuses so it won't have to change familiar patterns. Human beings are usually quite resistant to changing their habits. According to behavioral psychologists, *it takes twenty-one days of consistently repeating an activity before your mind accepts the activity as a habit.* (And Benjamin Franklin said that anything you do for twenty-one days will make or break a habit.) There are several steps you can take to ensure you'll stick with your new exercise program.

The first step is to choose an exercise program that includes activities you honestly like to do. Ideally you will choose a variety of sports, such as jogging, bicycling, swimming, and weight training, to work different muscle groups and give you a change of pace. Most important, though, is to choose an activity that you won't dread doing a minimum of three times a week.

Next, create an exercise plan that seems easy to accomplish. Perhaps you might want to make an agreement with yourself that every day you will spend thirty minutes jogging or walking, depending upon the way you feel that day. Or you might agree to spend fifteen minutes stretching every morning. Don't create a plan that requires you to be running ten miles a day, pressing 130 pounds on the leg press, and doing the splits within a month. Your mind and body will rebel against these drastic changes, and you won't succeed with any of them.

The final, and most important, step is this: you must resolve to stay with your agreement every day for twenty-one days. If you skip a day, you must begin the twenty-day cycle again. The reasoning behind this plan is simple. Because it takes twenty-one days to form a new habit, it will probably take twenty-one days for your mind and body to stop resisting the new pattern. Twenty-one days isn't a very long time, so if you find your mind coming up with excuses, you can regain control by reminding yourself that you only have to do it for twenty-one days. If, at the end of that time, you still don't enjoy the activity or feel you aren't receiving any benefit, you can always reevaluate. What you will almost surely find is that by the end of the twenty-one-day period, you no longer mind doing the exercise. It has become a normal part of your life. At this point you are ready to incorporate a slightly more demanding fitness program, still allowing yourself the twenty-one-day adjustment period.

The twenty-one-day process can be used in any area you choose. Later in this book you'll see how it can be used with your nutrition program.

Don't limit your visualizations to enhancing only your life. Expand your vision to incorporate our planet earth—filled with peace, love, and harmony. There is great power when many people visualize a common goal. An excellent example is the work being done by the Academy for Peace Research. The Academy for Peace

Research was founded to enhance world peace by promoting the awareness that individuals can play a part in creating peace.

The academy is now engaged in remarkable scientific research to test the hypothesis that people meditating together worldwide can bring about more harmonious conditions on Earth. Currently 3.5 million people have joined this effort and the results have been fantastic. (The study is available upon request; see the resource directory for the address.) I will share more about creating peace on Earth and what you can do—how you can truly make a difference—in the last chapter.

Start now and choose to live life the way you have imagined, without interfering with anyone else's right to do the same. When you advance confidently and boldly, with an excitement and enthusiasm about what you are doing—be it your job, your hobbies, your fitness program—then success begins to take hold. Whenever you embrace and celebrate what you are doing, success begins to chase you. You can't stop it and you can't escape it. You will start living your vision when you get out there and act "as if." Advance confidently in the direction of your dreams. Risk! This moment, commit to being the best you possible. There is power in commitment.

As Neville said, "Be still and know that you are that which you desire to be, and you will never have to search for it."

So follow your heart's desires. Commit to your dreams and regardless of appearances, don't give up. Persevere and you'll find the way to freedom.

From one of Paramahansa Yogananda's home study lessons comes the following story, which always helps me to continue on.

TWO FROGS IN TROUBLE

Once a big fat frog and a lively little frog were hopping along together when they had the misfortune to jump straight into a pail of fresh milk. They swam for hours and hours, hoping to get out somehow; but the sides of the pail were steep and slippery, and death seemed certain.

When the big frog was exhausted he lost courage. There seemed no hope of rescue. "Why keep struggling against the inevitable? I can't swim any longer," he moaned. "Keep on! Keep on!" urged the little frog, who was still circling the pail. So they went on for awhile. But the big frog decided it was no use. "Little brother, we may as well give up," he gasped. "I'm going to quit struggling."

Now only the little frog was left. He thought to himself, "Well, to give up is to be dead, so I will keep on swimming." Two more hours passed and the tiny legs of the determined little frog were almost paralyzed with exhaustion. It seemed as if he could not keep moving for another minute. But then he thought of his dead friend, and repeated, "To give up is to be meat for someone's table, so I'll keep on paddling until I die—if death is to come—but I will not cease trying—while there is life, there's hope!"

Intoxicated with determination, the little frog kept on, around and around and around the pail, chopping the milk into white waves. After awhile, just as he felt completely numb and thought he was about to drown, he suddenly felt something solid under him. To his astonishment, he saw that he was resting on a lump of butter which he had churned by his incessant paddling! And so the successful little frog leaped out of the milk pail to freedom.

For those who desire more information and support in affirmations and visualization, I have created an audiocassette called "How To Achieve Any Goal: The Magic of Creative Visualization/Living Your Vision." On side A I explain how creative visualization works, how to work with goals, and how to achieve those goals and live your vision—which includes peace on earth. On side B is a twenty-minute guided meditation that you can use every day to help transport you beyond your self-imposed limitations. You can use this tape daily to experience, in your own mind, your life exactly as you wish it to be. Other sources are the books *How You Can Use the Technique of Creative Imagination To See Your Dreams Come True,* by Roy Eugene Davis, and *Creative Visualization,* by Shakti Gawain.

Sample Affirmations

1. *I am in perfect health.*

2. *I love and accept myself completely, just as I am.*

3. *I eat foods that nourish my body.*

4. *When grocery shopping, I read labels and select foods with healthy ingredients.*

5. *My body is trim, fit, and beautifully shaped.*

6. *My muscles are firm and strong.*

7. *I weigh exactly what I desire, easily and effortlessly.*

8. *I know and accept that I can shape my body as I want.*

9. *I exercise regularly and vigorously and I love it!*

10. *I give thanks for increasing energy, confidence, and well-being.*

11. *My body is created to express health and wholeness. I hold this picture in my mind.*

12. *I am created to be healthy. I claim health and peace for myself now.*

13. *I dwell in love, peace, and confidence, with God as my source. I am now becoming all I was created to be.*

14. *Always the best for me.*

15. *This day I choose to spend in perfect peace.*

16. *The peace within permeates my entire being. I am joyously serene.*

17. *I live in the heart of God.*

18. *All my relationships are harmonious and wonderful.*

19. *I give myself permission to be healthy, happy, prosperous, and at peace.*

20. *I let God's light shine through me in everything I think, feel, say, and do.*

21. *Spirit is peace, the truth of my being.*

Following is a special meditation that you can use on your own, which will assist you in examining beliefs that have been standing in the way of you being, doing, and having all you truly desire and deserve. You can read through this on your own or have a friend read it to you as you meditate on it or you can get my tape called "Celebrate Your Magnificence," which includes this guided meditation. Use the meditation every day for twenty-one days in order to recognize and let go of negative conditioning and to recognize your magnificence. When I do this meditation in my workshops and seminars, I hear positive responses on how this helps to transform lives.

Let's begin now. Sit comfortably, with your back straight, and your eyes closed, breathing slowly and deeply for about three to five minutes. As you breathe, completely fill up your lungs, hold your breath for as long as is comfortable, then slowly let it out through slightly parted lips. Continue your deep breathing for a few moments while you completely relax.

Imagine that a wave of golden relaxation is entering all your toes. It's moving up the balls of your feet, into the arches, and up to the heels and ankles. It's completely relaxing, completely relaxing. And this golden relaxing power is now moving up your calves and into your knees, relaxing them completely. Now up your thighs and into your hips, just completely relaxing all the muscles and tendons. And this relaxing power continues to move up into the base of your spine. And it's relaxing your spine. Feel the relaxing

power m o v i n g s l o w l y u p y o u r s p i n e and into
the back of your neck and shoulders. The back of your neck and
your shoulders are now loose and limp. . .loose and limp. And this
relaxing power is now entering the upper arms at the same time.
And it's moving on into your forearms and hands. And your fingers
and hands and forearms and upper arms are now completely
relaxed. And this golden relaxing power is now moving up the back
of your neck and into your scalp, relaxing your scalp. And on up
now, into your facial muscles, relaxing your facial muscles. Your
eyes are relaxed, your jaw is relaxed, and your mouth, throat, and
tongue are relaxed. Your entire body is now relaxed all over and is
filled with a golden relaxing light that feels warm and comfortable,
all over, in every way. All tension is gone from your body and mind.
Continue to keep your eyes closed and breathe slowly and deeply.

Now imagine, very vividly, that you are walking down a forest
path. It is a beautiful, sunny day and the path feels so cool and
smooth beneath your bare feet. You are wearing very comfortable
clothes, and you carry nothing with you except an empty basket in
your hand. Walk down the forest path for a moment and soak up
the serenity and peace you feel within it. . .

As you are walking along, you notice something off to the right
side of the path. It seems strange, yet somehow all too familiar. It
is not a part of you, but it is something you're used to carrying with
you wherever you go. It is a belief you have about your own body
that is limiting you. Pick up the belief, just like you have before,
and put it in your basket. Notice how the belief is heavy in your
basket. You can feel the added weight of it tugging at your arm.
You're used to it, though, as you've been carrying this belief around
with you for years.

Begin to walk once again down the forest path. Your journey
isn't quite as carefree now, but you can manage. Look over to the
left of your path now. Isn't that another one of your negative beliefs
that has been limiting you? This one deals with relationships. You'd
better pick it up and put it in your basket. You don't want anyone
else stumbling across it in the forest. It certainly is a burden
though, isn't it? You have to walk slowly and carefully now, just to
balance the heavy weight of the basket.

Isn't it interesting how the forest hasn't changed at all, even though the heavy basket you're carrying is spoiling some of your pleasure in walking through this lovely place? The forest is the same delightful playground it's always been; only you have changed. You no longer have the freedom to enjoy it.

Continue to walk through the forest now. There's a bend in the path in front of you, and as you round it you come to a dead stop. Right in the middle of your path is the worst belief of all, the greatest fear, the one you've wanted to hide even from yourself. Don't try to avoid the belief; you've done that in the past but it continues to get in your way. Instead, accept that you have this belief about yourself. Own it. Take responsibility for it. Now pick it up and put it in your basket.

Your basket is quite heavy now. As long as you are carrying it you must measure every step. There's no room for spontaneity, for playfulness. You can only trudge ahead, step by step, never able to look ahead or behind for fear of losing your balance altogether.

Continue to walk now and as you walk you begin to hear the sounds of a brook babbling in the distance. It's such an inviting sound. Perhaps you can rest there and set down your basket for a moment. You're getting closer now. Begin to perceive clearly the sound of the water, the wet smells of the river banks. It's there in front of you and there's a beautiful bridge arching over the water. Walk up on the bridge, set your basket down beside you, and lean over the water. You can see your reflection staring back at you from below. It is you, yet it isn't. Stare into the water and see how beautiful you are when your vision isn't clouded by your own negative beliefs. Perceive your ultimate potential when you move past your self-imposed limitations. (Pause for thirty seconds.) This is what you have the potential to create.

The only thing standing between you and your ideal vision of yourself is time, space, and your own negative beliefs. So let's eliminate the most formidable barrier right now. Pick up the basket you've been carrying for so long. Once again notice how heavy it is. Now swing the basket over the edge of the bridge and drop it into the brook. Feel your own sense of elation as you watch the basket bob gently down the brook, taking with it all your insecurities and fears. You are a free person. Free to create your own reality. Free to become all that you were created to be.

Leave the bridge now and begin to walk along the riverbank in the opposite direction of the basket. Allow yourself to wade in the water and feel how good the smooth soil feels beneath your feet. Splash and play and relax now for a moment while we pause...

You're feeling so relaxed and so at ease...completely at peace with yourself and the world and everyone in it. And you feel like you'd just like to stretch out in the sun for awhile, so wade back over to the riverbank and find a nice, soft spot to lie down. Do this now.

As you lie by the river, allow yourself to create in your mind a fantasy that symbolizes your success from creating new, positive beliefs about your body and about your life. Visualize yourself as a healthy, loving, happy, and prosperous person. See your body in perfect health and shape. See yourself in relationships that support who you are as a loving, valuable, and worthwhile human being. It doesn't matter whether you choose to fantasize about one area of your life or several. What is important is that you become totally involved in the mental movie and feel the emotions of joy and satisfaction and gratitude. What is important to you? See yourself now being that way. Affirm it, envision it and accept that it's already a reality. Do this now for a few minutes.

You absolutely have the power and ability to make this fantasy your reality. You are unlimited in your potential to create any reality you desire. Right now, right this moment is a new life, a new beginning. As you let go of the past, you are able to create the present and future. You do have the power. And you never dream without the power to make it come true. Right now, where you are you don't need to judge by appearances, for as you change your consciousness and you accept the truth of your being, gradually and sometimes miraculously, your life is transformed. Miracles are a natural part of life. Expect and accept miracles in your life now. These messages have been communicated to every level of your body and mind.

Now slowly begin to stretch all the muscles in your body. Take a few long, deep breaths and after a few moments open your eyes and feel your serenity, joy, and peacefulness. You are a truly magnificent, lovable and special human being, and I support you in making all your dreams come true.

Self-Discovery Questions

1. *What are my goals in the following areas?*

    — *Relationships*

    — *Career*

    — *Financial*

    — *Fitness*

—Interests and Hobbies

—Health

—Spiritual

2. If I knew I couldn't fail, what would I change in my life?

Action Choices

1. *Following is my ideal vision of myself, which includes all areas of my life. If I were living my ideal life right now, what would my life be like, what would the world be like, and how would I feel?*

2. *Am I living this life now? If not, why not? What immediate changes can I make toward this goal?*

3. *Listed below are the words and phrases that I now choose to eliminate from my vocabulary.*

4. *My relationships can be more like what I want them to be, not by trying to change anyone else, but by changing my own thoughts and attitudes in the following ways.*

CHAPTER 4

CHOOSE

H E A L T H F U L
N U T R I T I O N

*"Let food be your medicine and medicine be
your food."*
*"Nature heals; the physician is only nature's
assistant."*

—*Hippocrates*

Let's now take a close look at another ingredient essential for vibrant health—nutrition, diet, the foods you eat. Do the foods you eat really have a direct relationship to your physical and mental health? You bet they do! In fact, according to a report by the Senate Select Committee on Nutrition and Human Needs, six of the ten leading causes of death in our nation are directly related to faulty diet. That actually should be a comforting statement in light of the fact that you are the one who chooses what you eat.

There are many different reasons for eating certain foods. Some people eat for taste; if they enjoy the taste, they care little about what the food contains or even what it is. Some people choose foods based on convenience only, living on TV dinners or canned foods. Others enjoy complicated gourmet dishes with rich sauces, and some will eat anything just as long as their hunger is satisfied.

But the most important reason for selecting any one food

should be nutrition. Food is our life support system. Without good, nutritious food, our life force wanes. If we let things go too far, disease sets in.

Can you imagine what the movie character E.T. thought when he visited this planet? Watching television, reading newspaper ads, and listening to the radio, he probably got the notion that we ate only processed foods, foods that were boxed, canned, or frozen. It might interest you to know that by age 16 a person has seen more than 600,000 commercials on TV. Think about how many of those are junk food ads. It's no wonder America has been programmed into thinking that all food is nutritious, no matter how it's prepared. The creative challenge we all face is to maximize the advantages and minimize the disadvantages of the age in which we live. This is certainly true when it comes to the foods we select.

Dr. William E. Connor of the University of Iowa told the Senate Committee on Nutrition and Human Needs that the vast majority of Americans eat too much food, contributing to a wide range of health problems. He and other scientists have also indicated that it's not only how much we eat, but also the kinds of food we eat.

Many people in our society eat large quantities of food while nutritionally starving to death. Chemicals such as bleaches, dyes, emulsifiers, homogenizers, hormones, hydrogen gas, preservatives, softeners, and shortenings help to decrease the natural vitamin content of many foods in addition to contributing little to your overall health. These chemicals are found in many food products.

A recent report states there are now more than 100,000 fast food outlets, and they sell $45 billion worth of food each year. According to Michael F. Jacobson, executive director of the Center for Science in the Public Interest, the foods served there "can be as pathogenic as any germ."

Everyone from government officials to health experts has agreed that we are eating too much fat, cholesterol, sodium, and sugar and too little fiber—and fast food restaurants are partly to blame. A typical American diet has been linked in medical studies to hypertension, stroke, heart disease, diabetes, cancer, and obesity in millions.

Let's look at a typical fast food meal—a cheeseburger, french fries, and a soft drink. This is basically composed of fat (up to 64 grams, which is more than anyone should eat in one day), cholesterol, sodium (some fast food meals contain as much as 1300 mg.) and sugar. It is also virtually devoid of any dietary fiber. Consider also that such things as yellow dye #5 (associated with allergic reactions), the cancer-promoting sodium nitrite, and other harmful additives are often present in fast foods, and you have a list of reasons why fast food restaurants are not a healthy choice.

Actually, when it comes to fast food, pay attention to the first word in the phrase, and when you pass one of these restaurants, simply fast until you can find some natural, life-giving food.

One thing you can do immediately that will have a positive effect on your health is to start reading labels when grocery shopping; it will be well worth your effort. As you shop, are you more likely to buy products that have words such as *natural* or *light* printed on the label? Food manufacturers know that consumers are becoming more interested in health. They have learned that products sell better when there's a suggestion of health or the year's most popular buzzword on the label. Like sports clothes and accessories, health foods have become trendy.

The word *natural* means "coming from nature." There are "natural" cereals, "natural" beer, "natural" potato chips, "natural" cookies, and "natural" crackers. Products claiming to be natural, however, often contain unhealthy additives and colorings. Natural foods are not necessarily always better or even healthy. Nature produces sugar, salt, and tobacco—but are they good for us?

Packaging can also be misleading. Printed in large letters across the front of many brands of breadstuffs, you'll see *natural* or *made with vegetable oil*. Then in tiny print you'll see *May contain lard, palm, or cottonseed oil*. These are saturated fats and have been proven to be unhealthy.

From the *Nutrition Action Newsletter*, which is available from the Center for Science in the Public Interest in Washington, D.C., I learned that currently many manufacturers are using the word *light* on their food packages. There are some facts about "light" products that you should know. Although the Food and Drug Administration (FDA) recommends that foods labeled light have one-third fewer calories, this is not always the case. *Light* can refer to other qualities. A light taco shell, for example, may be made with wheat flour, rather than cornmeal, but it contains the same number of calories. Light pancake mix may have no preservatives or artificial flavors or colors added. Now that is important. But it's not always possible to be sure what the word *light* on the label means.

The only way you can be sure you're getting a lower calorie product is if you see the words "low calorie" or "reduced calorie" on the label. These foods have to meet specific FDA requirements. ("Low-calorie" foods have no more than forty calories per serving. "Reduced calorie" products contain one-third fewer calories than a similar regular product.)

To determine whether any particular product is better for you, read the label carefully and compare the nutrient and calorie content with other similar items.

Just as important is noticing the order of the ingredients listed on the label; they are listed in descending order according to what percentage of the product they are. So if water is the first ingredient, the product contains more water than anything else. Avoid products that list sugar (it can be written in different ways, such as brown sugar, dextrose, corn syrup, turbinado, and so on), especially toward the beginning of the list.

When you get into the habit of selecting mostly fresh foods, you won't need to worry about labels. Also, if you shop at your local health food store, you will find products similar to what you buy at the supermarket but minus additives and other health-destroying elements. Added chemicals may enhance texture, color, shelf life, and flavor, but they detract from nutrition. Foods are often treated to increase their shelf life, not yours. A rule of thumb to help you select healthier foods is, If you can't pronounce it, don't buy it. Also stay away from sugar, salt, flavor enhancers, and artificial colors.

I have been blessed with many great teachers in my life and, at this time, I would like to acknowledge one of my favorite teachers in the area of nutrition. Her name is Joy Gross and she is the director of the Pawling Health Manor in Hyde Park, New York which offers excellent individualized programs for rejuvenating the body through nutrition, exercise, relaxation, fasting—a holistic approach to living fully. Thousands of people have benefited by her program and the best part is that she's a shining example of living healthfully. Joy lectures around the country on nutrition and has authored many books including *Thin Again*, which I highly recommend.

The body needs six nutrients on a regular basis for energy, organ function, food utilization, cell growth and repair, and just plain good health. These nutrients are carbohydrates, proteins, fats, minerals, vitamins, and water. These nutrients do more than maintain the healthy appearance of your hair, skin, nails, and eyes; they also keep your insides functioning as they should. Some people think that as long as they clean their nails, brush their hair, and wash behind their ears, they've done all they need to do. This is like keeping your car waxed but not concerning yourself with lubricating and tuning the engine.

When you start thinking of your body as the place where you live, it is easier to start selecting nutritious foods. A necessary requirement for healthy food selection is some knowledge about the body's needs and how you can supply them. Keep in mind that not only does every nutrient function independently according to the body's specific requirements, but optimum functioning of every nutrient depends upon the presence of every other essential nutrient. For example, vitamins, of which there are many, regulate our metabolism through enzyme systems. They act like spark plugs, keeping us tuned up and functioning at high performance. Yet as important as vitamins are, they can do little for you without minerals.

The best diet is one properly balanced in these six vital nutrients. The first three groups, carbohydrates, proteins, and fats, provide calories, which are units of heat or energy. Of these three, carbohydrates are the best source of energy because they digest quickly, so potential energy is transported to the muscles in the fastest time, and they provide water to the body when digested, functioning as a valuable secondary source of liquid to the perspiring exerciser. When broken down in digestion, carbohydrates are reduced into various sugars. Glucose is the most prevalent carbohydrate sugar; others include fructose (fruit sugar) and lactose (milk sugar).

Because complex carbohydrates should compose most of your diet, let's look at them more closely. At the beginning of the century, almost 40 percent of caloric intake in this country came from complex carbohydrates: fruits, vegetables, legumes (beans and peas), and whole grain products. Today little more than 20 percent does. This is because our fat and refined sugar consumption has risen completely out of proportion to what's best for our health. Americans eat nearly 100 pounds of sugar per person annually. Add to that 32 pounds of corn syrup and 8 pounds of saccharin, and you get 140 pounds of sweeteners per person per year!

Soft drinks (about 500 per person are drunk annually) account for 20 pounds of sugar alone, and that figure does not include sugar-filled fruit drinks. Candy accounts for 16 pounds, and ice cream, ice milk, and other dairy products, 30 pounds. Consumers also purchase about 30 pounds of sweeteners (mostly sucrose, or ordinary table sugar) in bags or bottles. Where does the rest come from? Catsup, hot dogs, pastries, cakes, and breads all contain sweeteners; so do many canned products. Again, read labels! Avoid foods that contain sugar whenever possible.

In setting up new dietary goals for the United States, the Senate Select Committee on Nutrition and Human Needs recommends a dramatic boost in the consumption of complex carbohydrates and natural sugar (such as you find in fruit) to up to more than 50 percent of your daily caloric intake. Personally, I see to it that I get 70 to 75 percent of my caloric intake from complex carbohydrates.

Probably some of you hear the word carbohydrate and think it means a fattening or unhealthy food. Not true. It is the lowest calorie source of the three energy foods. It has 4.1 calories per gram; protein has 4.3 calories per gram and fat has 9.3 calories per gram. A medium potato, which is an excellent, nutritious food, has around 90 calories. Yet it gets labeled as fattening because of the butter and sour cream that is piled on top.

Junk foods have also given carbohydrates a bad name. Foods such as soft drinks, cakes, jellies, candy, and other sweets made with sucrose contain little nourishment. The same is true of breads and pasta made with refined white flour. These are called empty calorie foods because they contribute little but calories to the diet.

Carbohydrates come to us as sugars, starches, and cellulose. Natural sugars are found primarily in fruits; starches are found in whole grains, legumes, and many vegetables; and cellulose, also known as fiber, is the undigestible portion of plants. It acts as an intestinal broom and is found in vegetables, fruits, and the outer cover of whole grains. You might be surprised to hear that more than half the people in the world stay healthy and slim on a high complex-carbohydrate diet because it is high in nutrients and fiber and low in calories.

Fiber in a diet is an essential part of vibrant health. It's only been in the past decade that fiber has been awarded a place of importance in nutrition, and has been medically recognized in terms of a special diet for some disease conditions. But years ago I remember my mother telling me that roughage was important for a good diet. To this day she still reminds me to have an apple daily. But as foods have become more processed and refined, fiber has been removed from more foods. The tide, however, has turned; these days fiber is often retained or even added.

British physician Denis Burkit, in his excellent book *Eat Right— To Stay Healthy and Enjoy Life More*, as well as in his journal reports and magazine articles, has stirred the interest of health professionals in both England and America. He has produced evidence that diseases common to industrialized society—cancers of the colon and rectum, diabetes, heart disease, gallstones, hemorrhoids, and intestinal diseases—are almost unknown among rural African people. The difference, he believes, is the fact that industrialized populations eat diets high in meat, fat, sugar, and refined products but low in whole grains, fruits, and vegetables. Africans, on the other hand, eat little meat or fat but large quantities of high-fiber vegetables, grains, and fruits, producing frequent and bulky bowel movements.

How much fiber do you need daily? About 40 grams. Our standard diet contains only 10 to 20 grams of fiber, indicating that most of us should double our fiber intake for better health. So consider boosting your diet with more fiber. Select more fresh foods—

fruits, figs, vegetables, sprouts, legumes and whole grains, such as millet, oats, quinoa and rice. The Ohsawa brand offers excellent, wholesome rice, with "Ohsawa Rose" being one of my favorites. (See Resource Directory.) It's great for the figure, the teeth, and your overall health. By the way, don't fall into the trap of thinking it really doesn't matter what you eat as long as you take fiber capsules every day. Research indicates that fiber's metabolic action is linked to its being an integral component of a food, so choose to eat more whole foods. The potato and apple, for example, have about 4 grams of fiber in each. Three-quarters cup of strawberries has 2.4 grams of fiber and one-half cup of white beans has 4.2 grams. The Center for Science in the Public Interest offers a guide listing various foods and their fiber content. For more information write them at the address given in the resource directory.

Keep in mind the following when increasing the fiber in your diet: (1) Aim for forty grams of fiber a day. (2) To give your system time to adjust, add fiber to your diet gradually. (3) Drink plenty of fluids with whole grain or bran foods. (4) Include fresh fruits and vegetables as well as brans, grains, and legumes to get a variety of different fibers. (5) Eat about 50 percent of your diet raw to increase the fiber; when cooking, lightly steam rather than boiling or pureeing. (6) Avoid high-fiber diet breads that contain cellulose; this is wood fiber and can be constipating. (7) Whenever possible, select *whole* foods—choose brown rice over white rice. Choose whole grain pastas and noodles over those made with refined white flour.

Just because natural carbohydrates should be the primary food in your diet doesn't mean that you should discount the importance of protein. Protein helps build new tissue (growth) and helps repair tissue (maintenance). Here is an example of the myth that just because a little bit of something is good for us, a lot is better. Americans eat too much protein. We're convinced that large quantities of protein are necessary to avoid protein deficiency. Not true, as most nutritionists are now quick to point out. The average American consumes much more protein than the body needs and more than the recommended daily allowance (RDA) for protein set by the National Academy of Sciences. In fact, scientists purposely set the RDA 30 percent above most people's requirements. They know that people naturally differ in their protein needs, so they inflate the average person's requirement to cover people with exceptionally high needs.

Who requires more protein? Contrary to popular belief, exercise does not increase the need for protein, with one minor exception. Body builders may use slightly more protein than usual to build muscle. It's really not that much more, however, and many body builders already eat more than enough protein to cover muscle-building needs. Women who are pregnant or breastfeeding do require additional protein. Because all foods contain protein, an increased calorie intake during pregnancy would contribute to meeting the additional needs. Research has also shown that people undergoing severe psychological strain (such as grief, fear, or nervousness) or severe physical stress (such as surgery, infection, fever, or burns) use more protein than usual. Also, people who don't eat enough calories will burn protein for energy, creating a protein deficit. Total protein loss is insignificant, however, unless the person is consuming less than 500 calories a day, a drastic diet that should be avoided for many health reasons.

Many people believe that vegetarians must combine certain foods to get enough protein. This is not true. I speak from personal experience, because I have been a vegetarian for more than fifteen years. You do not need to combine proteins if you are eating enough calories to maintain your weight, and are eating a diet high in natural carbohydrates and low in fat. There are populations around the world that eat only 4 percent of their total calories in protein, and this is all plant proteins. Yet they have no problems with protein deficiency. Protein deficiency is the last nutrition need you need be concerned about in this country. For more information on protein consumption and nutrition in general, some good books are *Diet for A New America*, by John Robbins, *Spiritual Nutrition* and *The Rainbow Diet*, by Gabriel Cousens, M.D., *Staying Healthy with the Seasons*, by Elson Haas, M.D., *Vibrant Health from Your Kitchen* and *Chlorella: Gem of the Orient*, both by Dr. Bernard Jensen (see Resource Directory), *The Pritikin Promise*, by Nathan Pritikin, *The Food Pharmacy*, by Jean Carper, *The Hippocrates Diet*, by Ann Wigmore, and magazines such as *Health Science*, *East West*, and *Vegetarian Times*.

For those of you eating a high-protein diet, read the following carefully. The body can't store excess protein, but it can remove nitrogen and convert the protein into fat. Furthermore, high-protein diets are often high in fat as well, increasing the risk of heart disease, stroke, and bowel, breast, and prostate cancer. People tend to think of foods such as eggs, dairy products, and meat as pure protein. In fact, at least half the calories in eggs, whole milk, cheese, and most cuts of beef come from fat, not protein. Excess protein also inhibits the body's ability to absorb calcium, which can lead to osteoporosis.

Finally, too much protein can have an aging effect. Before the protein in meat can be put to use it must go through a process called deamination, in which the nitrogen is removed from the molecules. These are reconstituted in a form the body can use. At the same time toxic by-products of animal protein—mainly urea and uric acid—must be excreted by the liver and kidneys. Digestion of plant protein is much easier on the body; there are virtually no deamination and no toxic by-products to be eliminated. So a diet that's too high in protein—especially complicated animal protein—can wear your system down and age you prematurely. The following are good vegetarian protein sources: nuts, beans, tofu, sunflower seeds, and sesame seeds. Also good are potatoes, sprouts, eggplant, bananas, carrots, tomatoes, and avocados.

If you are used to eating a lot of protein or a diet that includes animal products, I suggest that for twenty-one days you try a new way of eating. Let your diet center around fresh vegetables, fresh fruits, whole grains, legumes, sprouts, raw nuts (a small amount), and seeds. Stay away from beef because of its high fat content and concentrated protein. If you are not a vegetarian, you may want to include some fish. If you eat dairy products, select nonfat or low-fat milk, cottage cheese, and yogurt. After twenty-one days you will feel more energetic and more alive than you have in a long time. For more reading on vegetarian sources of protein and the efficacy of a vegetarian diet, I recommend *Health Science* magazine, *East West* magazine and *Vegetarian Times* magazine.

Speaking of fat, although our bodies need a small amount of fat, here is another example where more is not necessarily better.

Americans eat more than double the fat their bodies need, and the wrong type, at that. Too much fat and cholesterol is cited as being responsible for many diseases, including America's number one killer—heart disease. If your diet includes animal protein, you can be sure you are getting too much fat. Work on cutting down on the visible fat in your diet. If you eat meat choose cuts that are less marbled, and trim off any excess fat. Do not fry food. Stay away from oil in your cooking. If oil is used make sure it's fresh and cold-pressed, and do not heat it. Although it is important to limit your saturated fats (meat, dairy products, and so on), it is still imperative that you receive a precise balance of essential polyunsaturated fatty acids. Although essential fatty acids (EFAs) were first discovered more than fifty years ago, it is only recently that their importance has come to be fully appreciated.

EFAs are found in the membranes of every cell in the body, where they serve a structural function and help maintain normal cell elasticity. These substances, although required in large amounts, cannot be synthesized by the body. That is why they are called essential.

Just as important is the fact that EFAs in the cell membranes serve as stores from which prostaglandins are formed. Like EFAs, prostaglandins were first discovered about fifty years ago. Over the past decade they have been the subject of Nobel Prize-winning research. It is now generally accepted that prostaglandins play a vital role in regulating important body functions.

In humans three families of prostaglandins can be distinguished, each derived from a different fatty acid. Adequate levels of one particular fatty acid, gamma linolenic acid (GLA), must be present in the body to permit prostaglandin E1 synthesis, which is believed to be responsible for controlling several critical functions of the body. Prostaglandin E1 is formed in a step-by-step manner from gamma linolenic acid (GLA) and dihomogammalinolenic acid (DGLA). With the exception of human milk, which contains substantial quantities, very small amounts of these precursors are present in food. Another fatty acid, cislinoleic acid, is present in a number of polyunsaturated vegetable oils, such as sunflower oil and safflower oil, if they are cold-pressed and fresh.

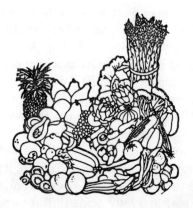

Until recently it was thought that the normal dietary intake of vegetable oils was sufficient to ensure most people adequate supplies of cislinoleic acid for production to prostaglandin E1. Recent studies, however, indicate that there may not be enough active EFAs in the average diet because of modern processing methods. Many oils are overprocessed and many have been found to be rancid. Our processed Western diet, which includes high levels of saturated fats, transfatty acids, and cholesterol, along with chronic alcohol intake, aging, diabetes, cancer, viral infection, ionizing radiation, zinc deficiency, and other factors inhibit the conversion of cislinoleic acid to gamma linolenic acid. Efamol brand Evening Primrose Oil is a good source of EFAs.

It's also been shown that the EFA content of human adipose tissue shows a highly significant negative correlation with arterial blood pressure. That is, the higher the EFA level, the lower the blood pressure. In preliminary studies on people with hypertension, evening primrose oil as a source of EFAs was considerably more effective in lowering blood pressure than higher doses of other polyunsaturates.

Although the EFAs are necessary for vibrant health, you must still keep your fat and cholesterol levels low. Two exceptional researchers received the Nobel Prize in medicine for their work in the area of cholesterol and lipid metabolism. The best-known work of Michael S. Brown, M.D., and Joseph L. Goldstein, M.D., of the

University of Texas Health Center at Dallas, involved the discovery of a component in each cell of the body called the low density lipoprotein (LDL) receptor, which is instrumental in regulating blood cholesterol levels. They found that these LDL receptors helped to physically remove cholesterol from the circulation into the cells, where the cholesterol was utilized for a variety of normal cell functions. Brown and Goldstein discovered that in persons with a genetic disease called familia hypercholesterolemia, these LDL receptors were either absent or defective. These individuals have tremendously elevated blood cholesterol levels and suffer from premature coronary heart disease as a result. In some of the most severe cases, myocardial infarction (heart attack) has occurred in individuals younger than age five.

Brown and Goldstein's work has helped to explain why diets very low in fat and cholesterol are typically so effective in reducing the blood cholesterol level. They found that diets high in fat and cholesterol actually decrease the number of LDL receptors in the liver, thereby reducing the efficiency of the liver in extracting cholesterol from the blood. They found that when changing to a diet low in fat and cholesterol, the liver responds by producing more LDL receptors. They, in turn, clear more cholesterol from the blood, thus reducing blood cholesterol levels. The Brown and Goldstein research provides evidence that strongly supports the nutrition guidelines presented in this book for the prevention and treatment of atherosclerosis and coronary heart disease.

Not all cholesterol is bad. In fact, cholesterol is an essential building block for cell membranes, nerve fiber coverings, Vitamin D, and sex hormones. But the body manufactures most of the cholesterol it needs, so any cholesterol-rich food we eat likely results in an excess. Current research suggests limiting cholesterol intake to 300 mg. a day, just 50 mg. more than the amount found in one egg. Most Americans eat twice that amount. The excess cholesterol causes a gradual accumulation of fatty deposits and connective tissue, known as plaque, along the walls of the blood vessels. Eventually, plaque build-up narrows arteries and reduces blood flow, increasing the risk of heart attack or stroke.

Cholesterol is manufactured in the liver. In order to circulate through the bloodstream, it is packaged in fatty protein wrappings called lipoproteins. The low-density lipoproteins (LDLs) distribute cholesterol throughout the body, dropping it off where needed. The liver also packages another type of cholesterol, called high-density lipoproteins (HDLs), which pick up circulating cholesterol and return it to the liver for reprocessing or excretion. The LDLs are the ones that build up in the walls of arteries and are tagged bad cholesterol.

Because of the high fat content of oil, I recommend that you limit your oil intake. Don't fry in oil and choose fresh, cold-pressed oil. Some recent studies found that olive oil, being a monosaturated oil, lowered only LDL cholesterol, leaving HDL alone. The polyunsaturated oils (safflower, sunflower, corn, and soybean oils) lowered both LDL and HDL.

When I use oil, say to make salad dressing (although I often make oil-less dressing), I choose extra-virgin olive oil, which are made from the first pressing. These oils are of a higher quality than the heat-extracted second or third pressing oils.

I also recommend that you limit your consumption of dairy products. They are clogging to your system. If you choose to eat them, select non-fat or low-fat products and purchase them raw and unsalted from a certified dairy, if possible.

One of my favorite foods, which composes almost one-quarter of my diet, is sprouts. Seeds and sprouts are one of the most potent sources of life. You can sprout the living seeds of certain vegetables, plants and grains, and legumes right in your own kitchen. It requires no soil: a jar or plastic container with holes in the lid is sufficient.

Growing sprouts requires little time and gives you the richest nutritional food value available. It is in seeds that nature has hidden the procreative powers that make possible the continuation of life on earth. Sprouts contain some nutritive values not found in the seed in its dry state. Vitamin and mineral content increases with the sprouting process. Here are some of the advantages of sprouting:

- *new crop of delicious food every two to five days*

- *no worry about soil conditions, weather, or bugs*

- *can be grown in any climate, any season*

- *simple to harvest*

- *fresh food that compares with meat in protein value*

- *compares with fresh fruit in vitamin C content*

- *has no waste*

- *excellent raw or cooked (although higher nutritional value raw)*

- *high in fiber*

- *one pound of seeds yields 6 to 8 pounds of sprouts*

- *can be used in an exciting array of delicious recipes, from dressing up a main dish to the main dish itself*

- *terrific in salads and in sandwiches in place of lettuce*

Alfalfa, mung bean, and wheat are probably the three most common sprouts, but that's just a start. I generally have at least a half-dozen different types of sprouts growing in my kitchen at once. Some of my favorites include cress, fenugreek, millet, lentil, garbanzo, peas, radish, rye, sesame, sunflower, corn, buckwheat, and red clover.

You can use a two-quart wide-mouthed canning jar with just the screw-type rim lid. You can then use cheesecloth to cover the mouth of the jar. Or most health food stores now carry complete sprouting kits, containing interchangeable screens, which may be used instead of cheesecloth. Such kits are inexpensive and are more convenient than cheesecloth.

How do you use them? Let's say you want to start with alfalfa sprouts. Put three tablespoons of organically grown alfalfa seeds in a two-quart jar. Fill the jar with bottled water, secure the mouth of the jar with cheesecloth and rim (or with screen and rim from kit), and let it stand for approximately eight hours. Then drain off the water and rinse the seeds thoroughly until the water becomes clear. Rest the jar on its side at a slight angle so that all excess water can drain off. Rinse two to three times a day, and keep the jar covered with a towel. On the fourth day remove the towel and set the jar in the sun for one day, allowing the sprouts to produce chlorophyll and turn green. The sprouts are now ready to eat. Remember to wash off any excess seed hulls before serving. Sprouts can be stored in an airtight container in the refrigerator for at least a week.

Different seeds require different soaking and sprouting times. On the following page is a sprouting guide to help you in sprouting your way to vibrant health.

Another nutritious food group you might want to consider adding to your dietary regime is sea vegetables. For many centuries people all over the world have harvested sea vegetables for use as food. In doing research for this book, I discovered that the Icelanders, Japanese, Native Americans, Hawaiians, Koreans, Chinese, Irish, British, Russian, Eskimos, and South Africans are just a few of the peoples who have traditionally eaten sea vegetables. The Japanese, who probably eat more sea vegetables than any other people, grade their sea vegetables for quality, just as the United States Department of Agriculture grades meat or dairy products.

The macrobiotic diet uses sea vegetables as an important element of its program. They are high in nutritional value. Dulse, for example, is thirty times richer in potassium than bananas are and has two hundred times the potency of beetroot when it comes to iron content. Nori, a brown sea vegetable that is sold in thin, rectangular sheets, rivals carrots in Vitamin A content and has twice the protein of some meats. Hijiki, a blue-black, spaghettilike sea vegetable, contains fourteen times more calcium than does whole milk. Sea vegetables contain Vitamins A, B_1 (thiamine), C, and E, and the all-important B_{12}, an essential compound that is rare in vegetarian diets but is needed by the body for healthy neuromuscular functioning and adequate iron. Sea vegetables also contain minerals.

Those of you who have never used sea vegetables before might want to start with trying them in soups or bean dishes or cooked

SPROUTING GUIDE

VARIETY OF SEED	SOAKING TIME (HOURS)	FULL WATER RINSE & DRAIN (PER DAY)	AVERAGE TIME TO HARVEST (DAYS)	SPECIAL HANDLING	SUGGESTED USES
Alfalfa	8	3	3-4	None	Juices, Salads, Sandwiches
Beets	8	3	3-5	None	Juices, Salads
Buckwheat	8	3	2-3	Remove remaining husks.	Juices, Pancakes, Salads
Chia	8	No	3-5	Mist	Casseroles, Salads, Sandwiches
Chinese Cabbage	8	3	3-4	None	Juices, Salads
Corn	8	3	2-4	None	Soups, Tortillas, Vegetable Casseroles, etc.
Cress	No	No	3-5	Mist gently with water 3 times a day or mix with other seeds.	Breads, Salads, Sandwiches
Dill	8	3	3-5	None	Juices, Salads, Sandwiches
Fenugreek	8	3	3-5	Mist gently with water.	Salads, Snacks
Flax	No	No	3-5	Mist gently with water 3 times a day or mix with other seeds	Juices, Salads
Garbanzo	8	3	3-4	None	Soups, Vegetable Casseroles
Lentil	8	3	2-4	None	Juices, Salads, Soups, Vegetable Casseroles, etc.
Millet	8	3	3-5	None	Juices, Salads, Soups, Vegetable Casseroles, etc.
Mung Bean	8	3	3-4	None	Omelets, Oriental Dishes, Salads, Snacks, Soups
Mustard	No	3	3-5	Mist gently with water 3 times a day or mix with other seeds.	Juices, Salads
Oats	8	3	2-3	Remove remaining husks.	Breads, Granola, Snacks
Peas, Alaskan	8	3	3-4	None	Omelets, Salads, Snacks, Soups
Peas, Special	8	3	3-4	None	Omelets, Salads, Snacks, Soups
Pichi Bean	8	3	3-4	None	Omelets, Oriental Dishes, Salads, Snacks, Soups
Porridge Pea	8	3	3-4	None	Omelets, Oriental Dishes, Salads, Snacks, Soups
Radish	8	3	3-4	None	Juices, Salads, Sandwiches
Red Clover	8	3	3-5	None	Juices, Salads, Sandwiches
Rye	8	3	2-3	None	Breads, Granola, Snacks
Sesame	8	3	2-3	None	Breads, Granola, Snacks
Soybean	24	3	3-5	Change soaking water every 8 hours	Casseroles, Oriental Dishes, Salads
Sunflower	8	3	3-5 (Green 5-7)	Remove remaining husks.	Salads, Snacks
Triticale	8	3	1-2	None	Breads, Granola, Pancakes, Snacks
Wheat	8	3	2 (Wheat Grass 5-7)	None	Breads, Granola, Pancakes, Snacks

SOURCE: *The Main Ingredients: Positive Thinking, Exercise & Diet*, Susan Smith Jones

with fresh vegetables. Recommended sea vegetables include agar-agar, arame, dulse, hijiki, Irish moss, kelp, kombu, nori, and wakame. Check at your health food store or a Japanese store for the best selection. For recipe ideas check any macrobiotic cookbook.

Overall then, concentrate on making the majority of your diet complex carbohydrates (such as whole grains and potatos), fruits, vegetables, sea vegetables, sprouts, and legumes, moderate in protein, and low in fat. What works best for me is a diet of approximately 75 percent carbohydrates, 15 percent protein, and 10 percent fat. I also eat around 70 percent of my food raw, so I get an ample supply of nutrients and enzymes.

Now, what if you are a serious athlete? How would this type of program affect your training? Very well indeed. Modern training programs for athletes stress complex carbohydrates.

It used to be thought that the more you physically exerted yourself, the greater your need for protein. We now know this to be untrue. Some of the country's most famous coaches and athletes have discovered that a diet consisting predominantly of complex carbohydrates provides almost three times the strength for endurance in athletic competition as a diet high in protein and low in carbohydrates. Dave Scott, one of the top athletes in the world, known for his triathlon accomplishments, is a vegetarian and follows the Pritikin diet. And I found that my high carbohydrate diet gave me plenty of energy for my Santa Barbara to Los Angeles run, a distance of one hundred miles.

A while ago I had a wonderful opportunity to work as a consultant for the Los Angeles City Fire Department. For thirty weeks I worked with the first group of women recruits. In the areas of motivation, holistic health, and particularly diet, I saw many of the concepts and principles discussed in this book come alive.

One of the female recruits usually ate a large breakfast, high in animal protein and fat. A typical morning meal consisted of two eggs, sausage or bacon, toast with butter and jam, milk, and coffee with cream and sugar. Although she didn't have a weight problem, by midmorning she was often short on energy and had difficulty in the endurance and strength aspects of her training. She also complained of an inability to think clearly for more than short periods. Within two weeks of changing her breakfast to more healthy, energy-promoting foods, however, she experienced an abundance of energy and increased mental clarity, important for participation in the rigorous training program.

What was her new breakfast, you ask? Her typical fare included fresh fruit and freshly squeezed juice, whole grain cereal and herb tea.

One of the other women ate too many dairy products—lots of cheese, milk, butter, sour cream, cottage cheese and ice cream. Other than that her diet was healthy, with an emphasis on complex carbohydrates and fresh foods. When she cut down on her dairy intake and began choosing more nondairy foods instead, she experienced a noticeable increase in energy. Even as soon as the third day on her new eating program, she was able to perform the endurance events, which included running, continuous stair climbing, and the fire hose pull, more easily.

Although most of us will never be asked to train as intensively as firefighters must, we can all make simple dietary choices that enhance our energy level, vitality, and mental clarity.

It's not only your physical health that is affected by what you eat. What you put in your mouth can also influence your mental health. According to Drs. Cheraskin and Ringsdorf, in their book *Psycho-Dietetics*, 80 percent to 90 percent of marital discord is due to nutritional imbalances. You may not totally agree with this statistic, but it is definitely worth pondering. In the family counseling I do, I am often amazed at the positive changes in behavior patterns and in how people relate to each other after making some basic changes in their diet. More specifically, I have noticed changes in interpersonal relationships attributed to a correction of blood sugar imbalances. Foods such as soft drinks, ice cream, candy, cookies, cake—all refined sugar or refined flour products, in fact—assault the pancreas. This organ will then produce too much insulin, causing blood sugar levels to plunge downward. The adrenal glands, known as the stress glands, which produce hormones that aid in returning low blood sugar to normal levels, react by growing fatigued, and the hypoglycemic individual experiences characteristic physical and mental exhaustion. Many people with this blood sugar imbalance show symptoms of irritability, violent temper, abnormal sensitivity, and extreme fatigue. One of the psychological conditions I have observed among people with blood sugar imbalances is extreme feelings of neediness. The continual emotional mood swings begin to alienate loved ones and create a vicious cycle, from neediness to unfulfilled expectation to rejection to neediness.

Poor eating habits also have a negative effect on children's health, behavior, and scholastic performance. Through his careful research the late Dr. Ben Feingold, a California allergy specialist, attributed allergies and abnormal behavior problems directly to diet. Specifically, he found an allergic brain reaction to a group of chemicals called salicylates. These chemicals are found in the flavoring and coloring agents used in more than 3000 convenience foods that are the mainstay of most children's diets. According to his research, the average child gets a poisonous daily dose of salicylates. The child starts the day with a loaded breakfast cereal, and by bedtime has swallowed untold amounts of soft drinks, fruitades, chocolate beverages, hot dogs, luncheon meats, and ice creams—a long list of familiar offenders. A conscientious parent unwittingly provides an extra dose when the child's daily vitamin pill is a brand that is artificially flavored.

Dr. Feingold duplicated a Jekyll-Hyde scenario by altering children's diets to either increase or decrease additives. When artificially colored and flavored foods were restricted, 60 percent of his patients calmed down practically overnight. Allowed back on such foods, they became hyperactive again. Miniscule amounts of offending substances can drastically alter a child's behavior. This is not surprising when you consider that the child's central nervous system is far more sensitive than is the average adult's. For more reading in the area of nutrition for children, I recommend *Feed Your Kids Right*, by Dr. Lendon Smith, and *Raising Your Family Naturally*, by Joy Gross.

Not only do foods affect your emotions and behavior, but they also influence your sexuality. Yes, unsatisfactory sexual relations yield to nutritional therapy. So-called aphrodisiacs are a multimillion dollar business, but are, in my opinion, a ripoff. There is really no one food to increase sexual desire or capacity. Rather, it is an aggregate of all the nutrients in the right combination, a good exercise program and high self-esteem that will assure a healthy body and mind and thus a healthy sex life.

Energy is another area that is highly correlated with eating habits. The better your diet, meaning a balance of all the nutrients the body requires, the more energy you will have. This principle is supported by Rob Krakovitz, M.D., author of *High Energy*. Thus, if you are concerned about your mental and physical health and you desire more energy, I recommend that you consider your diet carefully. Keep a seven-day diary of everything you eat and drink. Then examine the list, keeping in mind that it's not the food in your life that counts, but the life in your food. Foods that increase the likelihood of disease and promote fatigue must be avoided. That includes foods containing sugar, salt, white flour, hydrogenated fat, food preservatives such as the nitrates and nitrites, and artificial flavoring and coloring agents. By choosing your foods carefully, you can experience an abundance of energy.

Poor nutrition has been found to accelerate the aging process. As we age our immunocompetence (that is, our body's ability to defend itself against disease) decreases. Our basic line of defense against microbes or viruses or floating cancer cells is various white blood cells called lymphocytes. Some produce antibodies and others engulf the invaders. Also, certain nutrients—vitamins A (in the form of beta carotene), C, and E and the minerals selenium, zinc, copper, and iron—can increase the number of lymphocytes and improve their ability to fight disease. This fact was recently reported in *Nutrition and Immunity* by M. Eric Gershwin, M.D., and colleagues at the University of California, Davis.

Another aspect of the aging process involves free radicals. These are destructive chemicals found in some foods, such as rancid oils, and produced by cell metabolism within the body. Free radicals are thought to cause cancer and impair immunity. Again, certain nutrients, ones that act as antioxidants, or scavengers, can help by gobbling up the free radicals. The National Cancer Institute is currently doing a study to determine whether these antioxidants, including vitamins A, C, and E, and the mineral selenium, play a role in preventing cancer.

One of the best things you can do to retard the aging process is simply to eat smaller amounts of the highest quality foods available, according to two professors of pathology at UCLA. In a 1982 study published in *Science*, Richard Weindruch, Ph.D., and Roy L. Walford, M.D. (author of *Maximum Life Span*), reported that when the food of "middle-aged" mice was gradually restricted over a month period and then kept at that level, they lived an average of 10 percent longer than the control group. They also had fewer spontaneous cancers than control mice. Their conclusion and recommendation is to strive for "undernutrition without malnutrition." In other words, limit caloric intake while providing adequate amounts of all the necessary nutrients. It is not absolutely clear how dietary restriction slows down the aging process, but evidence points to its retarding the age-related decline in immune function.

One cardinal rule sums up what you need to know for better nutrition, slowing down the aging process, and increasing your energy: the less doctored foods you choose, the less likely it is that you'll need doctoring.

Sugar is one of the biggest offenders. It is a prominent factor in the development of overweight, diabetes, hypoglycemia, dental caries, periodontal disease, kidney stones, urinary infection, cardiovascular disease, intestinal cancer, diverticulosis, indigestion, hormone disorders, and mental disorders. In Helsinki, health officials have warned Finns that sugar is so dangerous that they would ban it as a food additive if it were newly discovered.

You're probably wondering what to use instead of sugar. My advice is to reeducate your taste buds gradually and accustom yourself to foods in their natural form. When I want a sweetener, I use Westbrae's Brown Rice Syrup, organic and traditional. Brown Rice Syrup contains complex sugars, rather than simple sugars. The more complex a sugar is, the more digestion is required before the body can use it. To replace the liquid sweeteners like corn syrup and honey in your recipes, substitute 1 for 1. To replace dry sweeteners like sugar and fructose, reduce liquid ingredients by one-fifth, then substitute 1 for 1. For centuries the fresh juice of maguey (ma-*gay*), known to the Mexican country people as aguamiel, was extracted from a plant and used as a food and as a tonic rich in many nutrients. It has a rich, exotic flavor, sort of a cross between honey and molasses. Both Brown Rice Syrup and Maguey are available in health food stores.

Do you ever salt your food before you taste it? Are you addicted to salt? Are you one of those who thinks food tastes bland without salt? If so, are you aware of the deleterious effects that too much sodium has on your health? Like sugar, salt seems to be ubiquitous in most processed foods. Most Americans ingest four or more times the salt that is needed by the body. In fact, you receive enough sodium in your food naturally and don't need to add any extra when cooking or eating. Too much salt has been linked with high blood pressure and water retention. Too much salt also affects your taste buds. Those of you who are used to salting everything will be surprised how wonderful and delicious unsalted foods really are. I'm not suggesting you never season anything. On the contrary, seasonings can truly enhance foods. I am recommending that you be selective and choose only those seasonings that support your health. Next time you are in a health food store, check out the saltless seasonings and herbs and experiment with them. The Parsley Patch brand offers a variety of saltless spice and herb blends, such as lemon pepper, Oriental, garlicsaltless, curry, all-purpose, French, spicy cinnamon, Italian and popcorn. The profits from popcorn blend go to a private Peace Corps in Kenya to buy medical supplies and build medical facilities.

Wherever possible, select fresh fruits and vegetables rather than frozen or canned. If you are unable to get the fresh produce you want, then choose frozen (without salt or sugar) over canned. Make sure you get a variety of green and yellow vegetables. One of my favorites is broccoli. Eating one cup of steamed broccoli gives you almost 800 percent of the United States Recommended Dietary Allowance (U.S. RDA) for vitamin A, more that 200 percent of the U.S. RDA for vitamin C, 13 percent for calcium, 9 percent for phosphorus and thiamine, 6 percent for niacin and iron, five grams of protein, six grams of fiber, and no cholesterol—all this for only fifty calories. The National Cancer Institute tells us that eating cruciferous (cabbage family) vegetables such as broccoli, cabbage, cauliflower, brussels sprouts, and turnips may reduce your risk of colon cancer.

Do you sometimes crave something crunchy? Raw vegetables are a great choice. Try broccoli raw with a dip or marinated in a lemon-herb dressing or simply steamed. Broccoli florets cook more quickly than stalks. So if you want to cook the stalk with the florets attached, peel the stem for even cooking. Use a vegetable peeler and begin peeling at the end closest to the floret. If you used only florets and have stalks left over, a nice way to prepare them is to cut them into one-quarter inch coins. These discs make a wonderful side dish or garnish for soup.

A word about juices. Choose only fresh juice, unheated. Consider purchasing a juicer. The Champion Juicer is an excellent all-around juicer, as it's easy to use and clean, makes high-quality juice, and can be used to make nut butters, grind grains (with an attachment), and make delicious non-dairy frozen desserts using only frozen fruit. There's no beverage better (with the exception of fresh water) than just-made fresh fruit or vegetable juice. **The Juiceman Juicer** is also excellent. I use it daily and take it with me when I travel.

Instead of drinking sugar-laden beverages, simply add some salt-free carbonated water to your fresh juice. This drink is far superior to any canned or bottled soda pop.

Don't forget that all-important nutrient, water. Without water we would die in a matter of days. It makes up 70 percent of the body, and is a necessary part of every body function. Because we need to drink so much water to help keep us healthy, it only seems good sense to select a pure, wholesome water.

I have never found any tap water that I like. Because water is such an essential part of my health regime, I usually carry a bottle of pure water with me. The best-tasting water I have found is called Volvic. It comes from France and is available in health food stores. It has the cleanest, lightest, freshest taste I have ever experienced. That's probably because it comes from the Auvergne Mountains of central France, from almost half a mile below the earth. The spring is protected by 17 square miles of mountain wilderness free of industry, intensive farming, or human habitation. Because of these exceptional geological and geographical conditions, Volvic is free of impurities. It is also low in mineral content and has a perfectly balanced pH value of 7.0, meaning that it is neither acid nor alkaline. Each day Volvic water is extracted at a depth of two hundred feet and is put into bottles there at the source, without contact with the air, so that it loses none of its properties.

Until I discovered this water at my local health food store, it was sometimes difficult to drink all the water that I knew my body needed. Now I look forward to each sip.

One delicious beverage you can make with pure, wholesome water is herb tea. I drink two cups of tea each day, one early in the morning and one at night before I go to bed. The herbs in many teas are soothing to the body, but you must be sure the tea you select is a healthy one, without any caffeine. Celestial Seasonings Herb teas are the ones I have used and recommended for years because of their high quality. I always have an assortment of tea bags in my purse, house, car, and office, so I'm never without this tea. Some of my favorites from Celestial Seasonings Herb teas include Almond Sunset, Cinnamon Rose, Cranberry Cove, and Raspberry Patch. Try them hot or cold. They're healthy and refreshing.

By now you have the basic information on which foods to eat and which to avoid for vibrant health. But just as important as choosing your foods carefully is eating moderately and simply.

Thirty years ago one of the biggest dietary problems facing Americans was nutritional deficiencies. Now the biggest problem is overconsumption. We eat much more food than our bodies need, and this adds pounds, extra stress, fatigue, and emotional problems. How much and what you eat affects your opinion of yourself, so eat to support your self-esteem. Start taking smaller portions and you'll find that you really do feel much better and have more energy.

My theory about overweight is that we eat too much (especially of the wrong kinds of foods) because some of our desires, longings, and goals are frustrated, *and* this frustration occurs because we have accepted false beliefs and ideas of personal unworthiness and don't believe we can achieve our goals. We have little self-confidence and our energies are directed toward sensual pleasure rather than toward achievement, acceptance, and service. Choose to make food an incidental part of your life by filling your life so full of meaningful things that you'll hardly have time to think about food.

Start with unconditional love and acceptance for yourself just the way you are. *Let yourself be loved.* As you love yourself you will then more easily and effortlessly treat your body lovingly by choosing healthy foods in smaller amounts, regular vigorous exercise, and positive thoughts and words.

What it all boils down to is this: eat to live, don't live to eat. First meet your body's physiological needs, rather than centering on your psychological needs. The more nutritious and health-giving the foods you eat, the less you will overeat, because your body will be satisfied on food that is abundant in nutritional value. Keep in mind this ancient Egyptian quote, "Most of what we eat is superfluous. Hence, we only live on one-quarter of all we swallow. Doctors live off the other three-quarters."

If you are currently on a diet, especially one that limits your calorie intake to less than 1000 a day and you're not under your doctor's supervision, I would encourage you to go off it. Diets just don't work. If they did, there wouldn't be so many new diet books out each year. I just read a report that more than 40 million Americans will try a new diet this year—and 95 percent will fail. I know people who have repeatedly tried fasting followed by sticking with a very low calorie intake daily. Now I am not against occasional fasting; it is an important part of a health program if it is carried out under the supervision of a health professional. But some people eat horrendously, then fast for a few days, then barely eat at all for a few days, to be followed again by another fast. This has a detrimental effect on one's body warmth and basal metabolic rate (BMR). The BMR is the energy required to keep you functioning; it regulates all the body functions, including breathing, cell growth and repair, and thinking. When you exercise regularly you increase the amount of muscle tissue and therefore increase your BMR, making it harder to put on weight.

But when you diet often, fast too frequently, and don't exercise regularly, your BMR decreases and you'll gain weight more easily. When you deprive your body of the calories it needs to function optimally, as a safeguard, your body responds by lowering its metabolism to conserve energy. At the same time your body may begin to burn its own protein mass (muscle) in order to meet its energy needs. As a result muscle is lost and metabolism is further lowered. To add to this descending spiral, due to lack of calories, you may experience a lack of energy, which further discourages you from exercise, simply because you feel too fatigued.

The solution is this: exercise on a regular basis, eat only wholesome foods without stuffing yourself, and never think or speak negatively about your body or yourself.

Losing weight begins first with how you feel about yourself. If you change your attitude about yourself, you will change your attitude about food. Eating will no longer be compulsive. You will begin to notice how food tastes. You will also begin to select natural, health-promoting, low-calorie foods, such as fresh fruits, fresh vegetables, whole grains, sprouts, legumes, and if you are not a vegetarian, fish.

Go to your kitchen cupboard and get rid of any food products that no longer serve your goal of being radiantly fit and healthy. List those products here:

Mixing too many different foods at one meal, especially rich foods, can be stressful for the body, especially the digestive system. You know how you feel after eating a large holiday meal. Heavy. Tired. Stuffed.

In my experience sensible food combining is an important principle to follow to increase energy, lose weight, and prevent intestinal gas and other digestive disorders. When you mix too many foods at one meal, it's hard to truly appreciate any one of them fully. Consider integrating monomeals into your eating program at least once a week. That means eating only one food at the meal. For example, have some fruit for breakfast, one kind, say oranges, and have as many as you want without stuffing yourself. You might choose to have two or three. Or for dinner you might select a bowl of brown rice or one or two baked potatoes. This way you give your digestive system a rest, you eat less food, and you really appreciate how good the food tastes. I incorporate monomeals into my nutrition program several times a week, and every so often I choose one food to have all day, such as fresh fruit. This is not a program you'll want to use every day, but on occasion it can definitely enhance your health and well-being.

Don't make a habit of eating late at night. It is best to eat the majority of your dietary intake before dark, if possible; Eating too close to bedtime can lead to both poor use of food and poor sleep.

By the way, eating foods with inadequate nutritional value can also have negative effects on the skin, according to Ole Henriksen's *Seven Day Skin Care Program: The Scandinavian Method for a Radiant Complexion*. In this enlightening book the author explains how to eat healthfully, and includes a seven-day menu and recipe program that fosters not only radiant skin but also overall vibrant health.

You may be wondering about supplements. I believe that supplements were not needed years ago. Today's edibles, however, grown on mineral-depleted soils, manufactured with an eye to appearance, and processed to last on store shelves, lose nutritional value every step of the way. As a result of technological manipulations, items formerly considered highly nutritious are hardly worth being called foods any longer. For example, there is a complete loss of vitamins and minerals in the manufacturing of white sugar. There's a loss of vitamin C in storing, in prolonged freezing, and in precooking of convenience foods. You can add to the list a loss of the essential fatty acids in the hydrogenation of fats and a loss of several nutrients, particularly vitamins B and E in the milling of grains. Take bread, for example. Many breads in today's supermarkets are high in nothing but refined carbohydrates. "But they're enriched," you say. "It says so right on the label." According to Earl Mindel, author of the best-selling *The Vitamin Bible*, twenty-two natural nutrients are removed and are replaced with three B vitamins, vitamin D, calcium, and iron salts. It hardly seems like a fair trade.

What is the effect of enriched grain products on health? Roger J. Williams, Ph.D., director of the Clayton Biochemical Foundation at the University of Texas, found that commercially enriched bread was so low in nutrients that of 64 laboratory rats fed nothing but the enriched bread, 40 died of malnutrition and the growth of the survivors was severely stunted.

Foods also run a nutritional obstacle course when they reach the kitchen. Heat is the greatest single nutrition wrecker. Many foods that have already been nutritionally wounded by being blanched, sterilized, dehydrated, pasteurized, toasted, smoked, puffed, or roasted are then cooked to death at home. Canned peas, for example, have lost 94 percent of their original value by the time they are eaten. The frozen variety lose 50 percent by the time they are thawed, and 83 percent by the time they are cooked and eaten. Even fresh peas lose 56 percent of their original vitamins during preparation.

In addition to the foods you eat, other factors create a deficiency of nutrients. These are stress-related factors such as anxiety, stress, pollution, noise, fumes, poor water—and the list goes on. Did you know that one cigarette destroys twenty-five mg. of vitamin C? Ten million American women take oral contraceptives, unaware that the pill can interfere with the availability of vitamin B_6, vitamin B_{12}, folic acid, and vitamin C? While under stress, whether physical or psychological, the body increases its use of vitamins, especially the B complex vitamins. These vitamins are required in greater amounts as they are essential for the optimal performance of adrenal hormones. The adrenal hormones, including cortisone, are part of our early defense against stress. When needed, the body will begin to produce them at elevated levels within seconds. If you ask the average physician where the body gets cortisone from, he or she will reply that it comes from either the adrenal glands or the pharmacist. Few physicians are aware that the chemical requirements for the body's manufacturing of cortisone include vitamin C, two B vitamins, pantothenic acid, and niacinamide. Supporting your own ability to make hormones to combat stress is not only safer than taking synthetic cortisone, it is biologically sound.

The concept that supplemental doses of certain nutrients can supply nutritional insurance and improve health in the face of an unfriendly environment is well established, and deserves consideration by everyone interested in health and living fully.

I receive countless letters each month asking about which food supplements I use, and when I lecture on nutrition, I am asked most often about supplements, what I recommend and what I take personally, so I'll discuss this here. I spend several hours weekly engaged in physical activity, and am tuned in to my body's needs and how various foods and food supplements affect my energy, performance, and well-being. Be aware, however, that inasmuch as we each have a different body and my way of life may not be the same as yours, what I require may be different from what you require. If you would like more information on any of the supplements I discuss, write the company directly (refer to the resource directory) instead of writing to me.

Nutrients are supplied, to a small extent, by the body itself, but mostly by the foods you eat and the supplements you take. When choosing dietary supplements, make sure they are from a company that is dedicated to fostering health. Make sure the supplement is fresh and doesn't include sugar, fillers, or artificial colorings. Most respectable companies now put the date on the bottle or package so that you can check for freshness. I have toured several vitamin company facilities to check on integrity before taking certain supplements. Recently, along with Drs. Lendon Smith and Robert Mendelsohn, I toured the plant of Naturally Vitamin Supplements in Scottsdale, Arizona. We were all impressed with the company's commitment to producing only the highest-quality products.

When taking supplements, remember to take them either during or following meals, for supplements are best utilized while the digestive juices are flowing. Also, having all the essential nutrients present in the digestive tract at the same time is a favorable condition for optimal growth, maintenance, and repair of the body.

One supplement I take is a liquid herbal yeast called Bio-Strath. I heard about it years ago from some of my athlete friends, who said it was fantastic and I should try it. I bought some and took it regularly for a couple months to monitor its effects on my exercise program and general health. Delighted with an increase in energy and a greater sense of well-being, I decided to do some more investigating. After reading hundreds of pages of studies done on this product, I was so impressed that I flew to Switzerland, where Bio-Strath is made, to learn even more.

Produced for more than thirty-five years and available in more than thirty-five countries, this liquid herbal yeast is rich in the cell energy molecule ATP as well as vitamins, amino acids, proteins RNA/DNA, minerals, and other enzymes the body needs to digest and metabolize foods.

The yeast is produced naturally through a patented process without heat treatment, artificial coloring, or artificial flavoring. Wild Candida utilis yeast is fed on a culture of organically grown herbs. Honey, malt, and orange juice are added to enhance flavor.

A plethora of supporting research stands behind this product. Studies carried out in medical centers around the world and published in some of the most authoritative medical journals demonstrate its effectiveness in helping the body assimilate and utilize nutrients from foods and helping to increase energy levels. Studies have also verified its nontoxic and nonallergenic qualities.

To make sure there is no misconception about yeast and your health, I would like to clarify a few points. In 1983, when Dr. Crook's book *The Yeast Connection* was first published, many health professionals indiscriminately advised against the use of any yeast product. No differentiation was made between the good yeasts and the bad yeasts. In fact, some yeasts, such as Candida albicans, are detrimental to human health and some, such as Candida utilis, which is found in Bio-Strath, are highly beneficial.

In Dr. Crook's latest edition of *The Yeast Connection,* he emphasizes the issue of good yeasts. The author also quotes John Rippon, Ph.D., of the University of Chicago, an authority on yeasts and molds, who says,

Not all yeasts contribute to yeast-related problems. Candida albicans...accounts for the vast variety of yeast-related health problems. On the other hand, Candida utilis yeast, the basic ingredient in the herbal yeast food supplement, Bio-Strath, has been used beneficially for 35 years in over 35 countries.

This is the only product ever endorsed by Robert S. Mendelsohn, M.D., pediatrician, lecturer, syndicated columnist, and author of many best-sellers, including *How to Raise a Healthy Child In Spite of Your Doctor* and *Confessions of a Medical Heretic.*

The best way to tell if this or any other product will benefit you personally is to try it. Bio-Strath, also available in tablet form, is available in your health food store and is distributed in the United States through Prince of Peace Enterprises, Inc. (See Resource Directory.) (If you would like to receive a copy of an article I wrote on this liquid herbal yeast, write the company.)

Chlorophyll is another supplement I take at least a couple times each day. Often referred to as nature's healer, chlorophyll has a wide range of therapeutic uses. It has been shown to enhance overall health by improving digestion, appetite, circulation, lung capacity and resistance to infection; it also aids in the body's use of oxygen and serves as an agent to stimulate metabolism. You will find this supplement in your health food store. I use Nature's Way chlorophyll liquid. I also drink fresh wheat grass juice regularly, and take Sun Chlorella (See Resource Directory) as they're both high in chlorophyll.

I regularly take a supplement to help keep my intestines healthy. The function of the human digestive system is to convert the food we eat into useful body fuel. A necessary and healthful contributor to a properly working digestive system is an abundant supply of the friendly bacteria known as Lactobacillus acidophilus. Although the word *bacteria* is usually associated with a disease or infection, it should be understood that there are many kinds of bacteria—some beneficial and some harmful. Lactobacillus acidophilus is one of the most beneficial to the body's normal functioning, and it helps maintain good health. I take Primodophilus.

Nearly two billion years old, Chlorella is a single-celled fresh water alga which contains a wealth of nutrients and health-building substances. It has been shown to be useful in the following: strengthening our immune systems; accelerating the healing of wounds, injuries and ulcers; helping to protect us against toxic pollutants; normalizing digestion and bowel function; stimulating growth and repair to tissues; retarding aging; protecting us against radiation. In *Chlorella: Gem of the Orient,* author Dr. Bernard Jensen says it's the highest source of chlorophyll of any land or sea plant. I use Sun Chlorella daily in tablets and granules.

Kyolic brand garlic, which is made in Japan is also part of my regimen. It is a purified garlic extract that affords all the benefits of garlic but leaves no breath odor. Perusal of numerous studies on this garlic supplement has shown me that it is effective in helping with sinus infections, bronchitis, influenza, and hemorrhoids. It also helps to rid the body of ozone and photochemical pollution caused by nitrous oxides; heavy-metal poisoning from lead, mercury and copper; chemicals, pesticides and waste fluids from contaminated food and water; and food additives, such as sodium cyclamates, which are absorbed into the bloodstream. I take Kyolic (liquid, tablets and capsules) as a general detoxifier every day.

For years I searched for the best multiple vitamin. Interestingly enough, my search led me back to where my nutrition education started with Adelle Davis. Years ago, Adelle had a powerful effect on me through her lectures on basic nutrition and her books (LET'S GET WELL, LET'S EAT RIGHT TO KEEP FIT). Two years ago I was pleasantly surprised to find that one of my favorite multiple vitamins on the market, ALL-1, was made by Nutritech, a company that had worked with Adelle Davis for over 35 years. All-1 is not a pill, tablet or capsule; it's a pure nutrient powder. Because All-1 is a powder, many of the problems commonly associated with huge multiple vitamin pills are eliminated (i.e. difficulty taking huge tablets or digestive problems). Additionally, since there are no binders, fillers, excipients, or additives, there are no allergic reactions with All-1. Best of all, because All-1 is a powder, studies show that over 96% of the nutrients actually reach a cellular level. One tablespoon of All-1, mixed in your morning glass of juice, provides 51 pure vitamins, minerals, and amino acids in a form that is enjoyable to take and easy for your body to absorb. ALL-1 is an important part of my daily nutrition program. (For more information, refer to the Resource Directory.)

What are your health goals? Would you like to have a slimmer, well-toned vibrantly alive body filled with healthfulness? Feeling better and looking marvelous will quickly compensate for the loss of dubious taste thrills of the past, such as fried chicken, white bread, ice cream, and potato chips. You'll find yourself looking forward to more healthful pleasures—the tastes of ripe papaya, luscious strawberries, blueberries, and ripe pineapple, sweet juicy grapes, a crisp garden salad, brown rice with steamed vegetables, and baked potatoes smothered in sauteed onions and mushrooms.

Your primary goal on this aliveness eating program is to get to the point where you are eating a minimum amount of the highest quality foods. Remember, the minimum is adequate! Euripides said, "Enough is abundance to the wise." You can put that slogan on your refrigerator door, over your mirror, and on your bathroom scale.

Although it's important to choose healthy foods, don't become a fanatic about what you eat. It's what you eat on a daily basis that makes the difference, not the occasional lapse. If you were to worry about every biteful that went into your mouth, I believe that would be more harmful than infrequent splurges.

Learn to think in terms of whole foods. It's when you begin cutting, cooking, and preserving foods that your system gets into trouble. Whenever you are able, eat your foods whole, just the way nature made them. Remember that nature has prepared them perfectly, complete with vitamins, minerals, enzymes, amino acids, natural sugars, fibers, and water, in the right proportions for efficient use by your body. Fresh fruits and vegetables, whole grains, legumes, nuts, and seeds—carefully selected and prepared to suit your particular needs and desires—are ideal foods for the vibrantly alive body.

You may feel that it's too difficult to switch all at once to a new nutritional program. That's a common reaction and that's okay. You can break in gradually if you wish, switching first to the foods that appeal to you the most and gradually adding the others. It may take a while for your digestive system to become accustomed to handling these new live foods.

Start by examining your eating habits and identifying those that are self-limiting. Some people I've worked with have had quite destructive eating habits. For example, one client grew up in a family that regularly served enormous portions of food. To this man, a normal dinner was a half-dozen pork chops, three baked potatoes, and several helpings of vegetables and bread. And this was after a day spent eating peanut butter sandwiches, milkshakes, and an array of candy.

In another case, when searching for the cause of her weight problem, one client recalled the childhood experience of hearing her mother repeatedly say, "Good girls always clean their plates." As a child she attempted to win her mother's love by cleaning her plate. At forty-two years of age, she was still "cleaning her plate"–and her mother had died ten years before. She had programmed her subconscious that to achieve love she must finish all her food, even if she wasn't hungry. The pattern continued in spite of her conscious desire to lose weight.

Right now your mind may also have some negative programming about your eating habits that will trip you up if you aren't careful. The mind will always choose immediate gratification over long-term satisfaction. The mind doesn't care if you achieve your long-term goal for a fit, lean, healthy body. You see, the mind wants you to feel good right now. It's important to realize that the mind isn't necessarily your friend. You must sometimes detach from it to achieve your long-term goals.

The question is how much to detach from your mind when it's insisting on that ice cream sundae. Here are some suggestions. First, acknowledge the power of conditioning; this I learned from one of my teachers, Eknath Easwaran. The difficulty in resisting sensory desire (whether for food or something else) comes from the force of conditioning. When a river has gained momentum it's hard to stop or even divert it. Most of our desires also flow in that way, along deep channels cut in the mind through repetition. Every time we are negatively conditioned, we lose a little of our freedom and our capacity to choose. So begin by becoming aware of what you are eating. Eating at the table, at mealtimes, and only when you are hungry helps, because you can more fully focus your attention on your food. When our attention is divided, we eat compulsively rather than from hunger. Automatic eating occurs frequently in front of the television set, or at the movie theater, parties, or sports events.

The entire process of eating needs to be given your full attention to get the maximum benefits. Be conscious of the hunger you feel before you eat; how the food looks and smells as you prepare it, serve it, and eat it; how the table setting looks; how the food tastes; the texture of the food; your chewing; your breathing; and how you feel while you are eating. Finally, after all this, be aware of and grateful for the feelings of lightness and high energy derived from the meal and the easy elimination of the food after it's digested. It's embracing this attitude about meals that enables you to appreciate simple, wholesome foods, and to eat less, feeling completely satisfied. Paying attention helps to develop the capacity to enjoy the simplest foods and to be truly healthy.

Stop eating just before you feel really full. In this way you are reprogramming your subconscious and are taking control rather than letting your habits control you. Stopping short of satiety helps you savor your food, and helps you to be free and in charge of your choices.

You begin the retraining of your senses by eliminating things that injure the body. None of us would drive into a service station and fill the gas tank with oil. For the car to run efficiently, we must use a particular type of gas, lubricant, coolant, and so on. When it comes to our bodies, we are often not so careful. We put in all kinds of things that nutritionists—and plain common sense—tell us impair the body's smooth functioning, just because they taste pleasant. We need to reestablish that the determinants of what we eat should be our body's needs, not merely the appeal of the senses. I have found meditating for a few minutes before each meal is a powerful tool that fosters choosing foods that promote health and harmony.

As you make a change in the foods you select, your food tastes will gradually change. This simple concept struck home the other day when a friend was telling me about a wonderful granola recipe she found in an old cookbook. I was surprised that an old cookbook would have the recipe she described to me, so I asked her what kind of cookbook it was. "Oh, a health food cookbook," she replied. "But you know, it's funny. I bought that book many years ago because it had this granola recipe. Because I love to cook, I took the time to glance through the other recipes. Although at the time I considered myself a natural foods cook, I was put off by the ingredients frequently used in the recipes, such as buckwheat flour, sprouts, and tofu. I thought those were fairly extreme foods, and I certainly didn't use them in my daily cooking, so I put the book on the top shelf and forgot all about it. Many years later I dragged it out to look for this granola recipe, and once again I began glancing through the other recipes. I couldn't believe how many delicious foods were described. It was then that I realized how much my tastes had changed over the years, and virtually without effort."

Pythagoras made the same point when he said, "Choose what is best; habit will soon render it agreeable and easy." It does seem that our taste buds change and adapt when we alter our eating habits, and the whole wheat bread that tasted heavy and grainy a few months ago may taste chewy and flavorful this month.

So understand how your mind works, examine your beliefs about food and yourself, exercise discipline and choice and, finally, make simple twenty-one-day agreements with yourself that start to create new habits, or programming, for your mind. The purpose of the agreement is to program new habits, new automatic behaviors that will help you achieve and maintain your ideal weight and high-level wellness. For example, some twenty-one-day agreements might be:

- *For twenty-one days I will gradually increase the fiber in my diet.*

- *For twenty-one days I will spend fifteen minutes each day imagining myself having achieved my ideal body shape and weight.*

- *For twenty-one days I will eat just to the point of fullness without being stuffed.*

- *For twenty-one days I will eat fresh fruit every day.*

These agreements each set up a new behavior pattern—one that works for you rather than against you. When you set up a twenty-one-day agreement to create a new behavior, you also create new beliefs about yourself. Making and keeping new agreements is an excellent way to positively program yourself.

Let's review some basic eating principles you've undoubtedly heard before but that bear repeating. The most important criterion for eating is whether you feel hungry. Don't eat just because the clock says it's time: eat only when hungry! Hunger is different from appetite. Appetite usually relates to the time of day. At 6:00 P.M. you automatically eat because it's dinner time. But food that's eaten without true hunger will not be utilized fully. Get in the habit of knowing when you are really hungry and satisfy your hunger then. Chew your food well so that it becomes a liquid that practically swallows itself. Chewing is the first stage of the digestive process. Chewed food is easier to digest, places less stress on the digestive system, and aids in preventing obesity. Your intestines, after all, have no teeth.

Eat your food slowly and deliberately. Be right in the moment with the delicious taste of your food. This will allow the digestive enzymes and the saliva to mix more completely with the food. Slow eating also gives your natural signals a chance to register, so that you can stop eating before you've gone past the point of being full; the signals of satiety register twenty minutes after fullness is reached. I eat most of my food with chopsticks, because they help me to eat slowly and chew more carefully.

Begin your meals with a raw food, even if it's only a couple of bites. Research shows this simple practice improves digestion.

Get out of the habit of drinking right before or during your meals; liquids dilute digestive juices and thus impede digestion. Be sure the liquids you drink in between meals are not excessively cold or hot. And kick the coffee habit; coffee is a health-destroyer. Did you know that 145 billion cups of coffee are consumed annually in the United States, mostly at breakfast. Let go of your attachment to coffee today.

Leave the table before you are full. Even when you feel that you could handle some more...stop. The body can handle only a certain amount of food at one sitting and anything over that amount creates added weight and stresses your body system.

Make your snacks primarily fresh fruits or vegetables, as they are easy to digest, supply roughage, and are low in calories. Have monofood snacks; eat only one food at a sitting.

Invest in a good cookware set. I recommend stainless steel because of its unsurpassed heating efficiency, durability and beauty. The brand I use is by Lifetime because of its exclusive 6-ply construction and lifetime guarantee. (Refer to Resource Directory.)

Finally, enjoy your meals. Sit down and eat without rushing or discussing problems. Appreciate and give thanks for the beautiful food and nourishment that you are receiving. Being in a hurry or upset or tired interferes with digestion and utilization of the food. Create an environment that's conducive to your getting the most from your food. These ideas became very important to me after spending time at the wonderful spa called Cal-a-Vie in Vista, CA. (refer to Resource Directory) Nutritionist Yvonne Nienstadt and Chef Rosie emphasize that it's not simply the quality of your food and the way it's prepared. Equally important is how it looks on your plate and how you feel when eating the food. When you eat in a healthy, harmonious way, your whole body is uplifted and enriched – physically, mentally and spiritually.

I have a program that I'd like you to try (after, of course, you receive your physician's okay). Over the next twenty-one days, follow as closely as possible the principles presented in this chapter, as briefly outlined in the following rejuvenation program. Before you begin, jot down any comments, key words, or phrases – whatever comes to your mind – regarding your diet and how you feel. At the end of the twenty-one days, write down your feelings again on another sheet. (Don't worry about spelling, punctuation, or grammar – just write down what comes to mind.) Read both sets of comments and see what comparisons you can make and conclusions you can reach.

TWENTY-ONE DAY REJUVENATION PROGRAM

Eliminate all:

1. *Meat and chicken (if you eat fish, do so sparingly—salmon is a good choice)*

2. *Dairy products (if you prefer, a very small amount of nonfat dairy products is okay)*

3. *Foods made with white sugar or white flour*

4. *Fried foods*

5. *Preservatives or additives, Junk food, and extra salt*

6. *Colas, Soda pop, Coffee or caffeinated teas*

7. *Liquids with your meals*

8. *All alcoholic beverages*

Emphasize:

1. *Raw food, 50 percent or more of your diet each day*

2. *Fresh fruits, vegetables, whole grains, legumes, sprouts, seeds, and nuts*

3. *Lots of fiber foods (gradually increase)*

4. *Pure water, at least 8 glasses each day*

5. *Eating less*

6. *Chewing all food well*

7. *Being grateful for your wonderful food and health*

8. *All the guidelines suggested in this chapter*

Rather than limit you to a strict dietary regime for twenty-one days, I'd prefer for you to select those foods you enjoy, as long as they fit into the healthy guidelines. What you'll discover after twenty-one days is more energy, a lighter feeling, more confidence, increased self-esteem, and a healthier attitude about food. Because of how vibrantly alive you'll feel as a result of this program, it will be easy to continue on with your new health-promoting nutrition program.

Here's a sample menu for a day. Upon arising, have a large glass of warm water with the juice of one-half lemon and a tablespoon of liquid chlorophyll. Then have some freshly made fruit juice. For breakfast, how about a bowl of fresh fruit. If you desire more than this, wait at least one-half hour and have some whole grain cereal, either hot or cold, or perhaps a bran muffin or other whole grain muffin.

For lunch you could have a sandwich on whole grain bread that includes a generous portion of sprouts. Try pocket bread and put all those yummy ingredients you would put into a salad. Or maybe you could have some hot, wholesome soup and whole grain bread.

For snacks, whether midmorning, late afternoon, or after dinner, try herb tea, fresh juice, fresh fruit or raw vegetables.

For dinner, how about a large raw vegetable salad with romaine lettuce, sprouts, tomatoes, celery, carrots, beets, mushrooms, bell peppers, and green onions. Along with the salad, have a baked potato with sauteed mushrooms, red onion, and broccoli. If not a potato, how about a bowl of brown rice mixed with your favorite vegetables or some whole grain pasta.

Read some books and magazines on health. Some magazines that offer excellent information on nutrition along with fantastic recipes are *Health Science, Vegeterian Times, Let's Live,* and *East West.* And follow your intuition and body's communication. Your body is always communicating with you. Listen to it and then follow your inner guidance. If you do, I am confident that you will soon discover what it means to feel vibrantly alive and full of health and well-being.

For more information on nutrition, please refer to my audiocassette "Nutrition for Aliveness."

Self-Discovery Questions

1. *What foods do I need to eliminate from my diet because they don't support my health?*

2. *What are ways I have been treating myself lovelessly through my eating behaviors?*

3. *How can I change the way I prepare food that will support increased well-being?*

4. *What beliefs do I hold about food that are sabotaging my health-fulness?*

Action Choices

1. *For twenty-one days I will eliminate the following from my diet and add the following to my diet:*

2. *This is the book, magazine, or tape I will use to assist me in my health program right now.*

   These are others I will use in the near future.

3. *Listed here are some supplements that I now choose to include in my nutritional program to enhance my health.*

4. *Following are at least five affirmations that support my being vibrantly healthy.*

5. *Listed below are the foods I have normally eaten that I know are not healthy and will eliminate on my 21-Day Rejuvenation Program.*

6. *Each day I choose to spend at least ten minutes visualizing myself as a healthy, radiant being who treats himself or herself respectfully and lovingly. (Describe in a paragraph how this vision appears to you.)*

CHAPTER 5

CHOOSE TO

B E F I T

*Walk your dog every day, whether you have a
dog or not.*
—Paul Dudley White, M.D.

*The health of the people is really the founda-
tion upon which all their happiness and all
their powers as a state depend.*
—Benjamin Disraeli

Americans' attitude toward fitness has changed dramatically in
the past thirty years. In the late 1950s regular exercise beyond high
school and college sports was almost unheard of. Today fitness programs are the topic of many a party conversation. Why the surge
of interest in exercise? I think it started out as a fad. Being a runner
or a weight-lifter or a swimmer became fashionable. Madison Avenue sold us on fitness. Well, great! One result of the mass marketing of fitness has been the development of truly advanced sports
accessories such as finely designed running shoes, slippery swim
suits, and more protective ski equipment. Most important, there is
an increased awareness of holistic health principles and the importance of a balanced way of life.

In California, which is highly body-conscious, the first thing
you might be asked when you meet someone is, "Have you got a
good gym?" I wouldn't be surprised to start seeing ads in the per-

sonal columns that read something like this: "Fit, trim female bodybuilder who bench presses 150 pounds and has a cholesterol level of 160 looking for a tan, strong, and toned man who has completed at least a dozen triathalons and has a triglyceride level of 75."

More and more people are beginning to see that beyond the fashionable aspects of fitness are many reasons why it's desirable to stay in good shape. Following a good exercise program will reward you with a better toned and more agile body, a heart that pumps more efficiently, and a less stressed body (without the negative side effects of drugs or alcohol).

Let's examine some of the ways in which regular exercise will benefit you—body, mind, and spirit.

Because I believe that a positive, relaxed attitude is one of the main ingredients for aliveness, I'll begin with some of the psychological benefits of exercise that contribute to a healthier attitude.

Exercise physiologists and medical researchers are discovering that our sense of happiness and well-being is greatly influenced by the presence of certain chemicals and hormones in the bloodstream. Brisk exercise stimulates the production of two chemicals—norepinephrine and enkephalin—that are known to lift spirits.

A well-respected British medical team, headed by Malcolm Carruthers, M.D., spent four years studying the effect of norepinephrine on two hundred people. Their conclusions:

> We believe that most people could ban the blues with a simple, vigorous 10-minute exercise session three times a week. . . . Ten minutes of exercise will double the body's level of this depression-destroying hormone—and the effect is long lasting. Norepinephrine would seem from our research to be the chemical key to happiness.

Another fascinating area of study is on endorphins and their effects on mental well-being. Since these morphinelike chemicals were identified a decade ago, they have been credited with serving as the body's natural opiate, helping us deal with pain and producing feelings of euphoria—the "runner's high."

According to Daniel Carr, M.D., a research endocrinologist at Massachusetts General Hospital, there is a more than 145 percent rise in endorphins during one hour of vigorous exercise. When studying a group of women, he found this dramatic increase even in those already in top physical shape. Endorphins are a potent key to a positive mood and an increase in pain tolerance. It is fascinating to ponder the idea that the better shape one is in, the higher levels of them the body appears to release.

Another chemical that lifts your spirits naturally is enkephalin, a chemical produced in the brain during vigorous aerobic exercise. Dr. William Glasser worked with long-distance runners in an attempt to understand the so-called runner's high. In his book *Positive Addiction*, Glasser credits enkephalins as being the source of that feeling. He says that the chemical composition of enkephalin is similar to that of heroin, and so is the effect (but without the problems). Long-distance runners can become positively addicted to the feelings of euphoria and personal power that result from the release of enkephalin. You can bet they look forward to their daily workouts.

This internally manufactured opiate, enkephalin, is also released into the system when you move from left brain activity to right brain activity, that is, move from ordinary consciousness into an altered state. Every process within the brain triggers, and is triggered by, chemicals. An altered state of consciousness (refer to Chapter 3, on visualization, for more details) feels good and is beneficial. This accounts for much of the popularity of meditation, self-hypnosis, jogging, brisk walking, and running: all are activities that cause you to shift from left brain activity to right brain activity which, in turn, causes the release of enkephalin. (For more reading on the brain, mind, and body connection, I recommend the newsletter *Brain/Mind Bulletin*, edited by Marilyn Ferguson. You'll find the address in the resource directory.)

Research also abounds in how exercise can work in conjunction with classical psychotherapy. Dr. Robert Conroy, M.D., of the Menninger Clinic in Topeka, Kansas, conducted a study that showed that exercise has a definite positive effect on depression. "It's not a panacea, but it is a useful adjunct for treating depression," says

Conroy. As depression becomes as widespread as the common cold, exercise takes on an even greater therapeutic importance.

So clearly, in the same way that a sedentary way of life negatively affects physical well-being, so too does it have a negative impact on mental health. Anxiety, tension, depression, and insomnia can be traced to a lowered level of activity—and respond therapeutically to a well-balanced increase in activity.

The problems of anxiety, tension, and depression are being addressed by Roy J. Shepard, M.D., Ph.D., director of the School of Physical and Health Education and professor of applied physiology at the University of Toronto. He feels that physical activity can enhance the quality of life. As such, his work focuses on the effects of exercise on the brain and the resultant good feelings.

"One of the main advantages is as an arousing stimulus. Quite frankly, it wakes you up. Also it improves your mood. Not enough stimulation makes you bored, makes you feel unhappy, miserable," Dr. Shepard says. In his book *Exercise Physiology and Biochemistry*, Dr. Shepard describes the underlying physiological processes associated with exercise. In essence, he states that the chemical arousal depends on the level of activity in the reverberating neuronal circuits of the reticular formation, a specialized part of the brain. So if neuronal activity is insufficient, a person feels bored, tired, and even depressed. Further, body movement also stimulates the muscle and joint proprioceptors as well, also increasing the activity within the neural circuits. The goal is to establish a personal exercise program that helps the individual stay at his or her peak level.

Much energy is expended in obtaining a fit body, but the rewards are well worth it. Many psychological and physical problems can be traced to a negative self-image, to an individual's dislike of himself or herself. Part of this self-defeating attitude can be sparked by inadequate exercise.

Conversely, one of Dr. Robert Conroy's hypotheses is that exercise has a beneficial effect on self-image, thus creating a better attitude. This happens, he feels, because exercise changes an individual's world stance from that of passive bystander to active participant. As such, each one of us can have control over our health and the quality of our life.

Dr. Shepard agrees. "One of the longer term benefits from exercise is an improved figure, posture and energy level, all having a positive effect on self-concept."

Another benefit of regular exercise is that the more energy you put into it, the more energy you get out of it. Unfortunately, the reverse is also true; those who are laid up for a period of time quickly lose wind and stamina, become easily fatigued, and experience the atrophy of muscles.

According to Dr. Lawrence Lamb, cardiologist and consultant to the President's Council on Physical Fitness and Sports, part of the reason inactivity leads to fatigue has to do with the way we store adrenalin. Lamb reports, "Activity uses up adrenalin. If it isn't used, adrenalin saps energy and decreases the efficiency of the heart." Thus the downward spiral of energy you feel at the end of a workday will only be worsened if you come home and collapse in an easy chair. "Exercise will get the metabolic machinery out of inertia," says Dr. Lamb, "and you'll be refreshed and ready to go."

Another work-related symptom that can be eliminated with exercise is tension. University of Southern California's exercise physiology laboratory director, Herbert de Vries, states that a single dose of exercise works better than tranquilizers as a muscle relaxant among persons with symptoms of anxiety tension—without, of course, undesirable side effects.

In a classic study of tense and anxious persons, de Vries administered a four hundred-milligram dose of meprobamate, the main ingredient in many tranquilizers, to a group of patients. Another day he had the same group of patients take a walk vigorous enough to raise their heart rates above one hundred beats per minute.

Over a period of time the doctors measured the patients' tension levels with an EMG machine to monitor the amount of electrical activity in the patients' muscles, because, as de Vries explains, "Measuring electrical activity in muscles is the most objective way to measure a person's nervousness." The results of the study were conclusive. What de Vries found was that after exercise, the electrical activity was 20 percent less than the patients' normal rate. Yet the same patients showed little difference after being given a dose of meprobamate. According to de Vries, "Movement is strong medicine."

Dr. Martin Cohn, M.D., chief of the Sleep Disorders Clinic at Sinai Hospital in Miami, agrees. "Exercise helps you deal with tension and provides a healthy release," he says. "And this is the key to a good night's sleep, a necessary component of mental well-being."

One of the body's nonspecific responses to stress is to release catecholamines. It has been found that exercise not only reduces nervous anxiety but also reduces the amount of catecholamines. In *Medical World News* it was reported that "an important benefit of physical exercise is the diminishing of excess catechols."

"Chronic tension states," say Drs. Paul Insel and Walton Roth of the Stanford University Medical Center, "are known to be associated with numerous bodily malfunctions such as ulcers, migraine headaches, asthma, skin eruptions, high blood pressure and even heart disease." The symptoms on the psychological side are no prettier. "Irritability, touchiness, moodiness, and depression, to name a few." Running, the doctors say, "has been shown to relieve some of these symptoms. Running does this by pulling the plug on pent-up tension."

Dr. William P. Morgan of the University of Wisconsin tested the lactate theory—the idea that exercise negatively alters the body's chemical balance, thus making it more tense. He found that lactate released by exercise differed significantly from the chemical substance that had been injected into anxious patients, and that exercise-induced chemical changes led to a "definite decrease in anxiety levels in normal and neurotic individuals of both sexes."

Most researchers point to the need for aerobic activity in order to produce truly beneficial psychological and biochemical changes. This is also true for cardiovascular improvements. This is why the emphasis is placed on running, jogging, brisk walking, swimming, aerobic dance, rowing, cross-country skiing, and other forms of aerobics. These vigorous, rhythmic activities appear to send messages to the brain as well as the endocrine system to shape up and feel good.

How often are we presented with a means to take control of our psychological and physical well-being through something as enjoyable and rewarding as exercise? The message is clear. A well-designed physical fitness program can add years of fulfilling, vibrant health. (And that knowledge alone has a potent positive effect on mental well-being.)

In my seminars I am often asked to suggest ways to improve the memory. Well, I've got the perfect answer. Exercise! Utah researchers studying the connection between exercise and various brain functions found that when people participated in a regular fitness program, both short-term memory and the ability to reason improved greatly. The researchers put a group of out-of-shape people between the ages of fifty-five and seventy on a four-month program of brisk walking. As a result of the increased exercise, the participants showed an enhanced ability to remember sequences of numbers and to use abstract thinking in correctly matching numbers and symbols.

Dr. Robert Dustman of the Salt Lake City Veterans Administration Hospital said, "I was surprised at the amount of improvement we saw. We expected to see some results in some people, but we didn't think it would be across the board." His further comment was that the brain seems to benefit from exercise because of increased oxygen transport, which improves brain function.

Not surprisingly, although the stress of exercise seems to enhance memory, work-related stress seems to have the opposite effect. You've probably experienced hectic, frustrating days at the office when you could barely remember why you were working so hard.

Now, if it seems as though exercise can improve almost every aspect of your psychological well-being, it can. But that's only part of the story. As discussed in the material that follows, regular aerobic exercise can also have a positive influence on many of America's most common disorders: colds, constipation, poor circulation, high blood pressure, excess weight, and low back problems.

Exercise may help prevent colds and infections. Dr. Harvey Simon, a specialist in infectious diseases at the Massachusetts General Hospital and a member of the Harvard Cardiovascular Health Center, says that white blood cells help the body fight infection, and that the type maintaining the front line of defense against infection enters the bloodstream as a result of exercising. According to Dr. Simon, aerobic exercise is at least potentially beneficial in warding off infection. White cells produce an agent known as pyrogen that stimulates body temperature to rise. Two studies have shown that exercise raises pyrogen output. This same substance also enhances certain of the body's immune responses. By introducing a transient feverlike state, exercise conceivably could help combat infection.

Constipation has become such a problem that many people regard it as normal. Exercise helps prevent and remedy constipation.

Aerobic exercise also improves circulation by increasing the number of vessels through which the blood flows. This has three benefits: it increases perspiration, which is an effective means of releasing toxins through the skin; it lowers blood pressure; and it helps diminish or prevent varicose veins. According to Dr. Robert May, a specialist in surgery and circulatory problems at the university in Innsbruck, Austria, "A brisk 15-minute walk taken four times a week is the indispensable minimum to get the calf muscles to force blood that collects in varicose veins back to the heart."

We've all heard that to lose weight you must consume fewer calories and exercise more. Although the logic is obvious, it isn't very encouraging. What is motivating is to know that exercise alters your body chemistry, speeding up the sluggish metabolism that made you overweight in the first place. Your body will become more efficient at converting the chemical energy of food into the heat and mechanical energy of work and you won't store as much of it as fat.

True weight loss cannot be achieved just by taking pills or reducing food intake. You might lose weight according to the scale, but you'll also lose your essential tissue, along with your good health. Effective weight loss can be achieved *only* through a balanced combination of a healthy diet, an effective exercise program, and, of course, a positive mental attitude. This combination is unbeatable.

Moreover, lack of physical activity may be a more significant factor in becoming overweight than overeating. In one study of 350 obese people, the onset of obesity was related to inactivity in nearly 70 percent of the cases; in only 3.2 percent of the cases was weight gain solely the result of increased food intake.

Regular exercise not only uses up fat reserves, it also works to tone and firm muscles and increase muscle-to-fat ratio. The value of this has been confirmed by two doctors who supervised a study on diet and exercise. Twenty-five women created a five hundred-calorie-per-day deficit through diet, exercise, or a combination of the two. Results showed that all the women lost similar amounts of weight, but those who exercised during the period of the diet lost more fat and less muscle tissue. Those who lost weight by diet alone lost less fat and more muscle tissue.

Nonetheless, the notion that you must run thirty-five miles to burn up one pound might discourage even the stoic from using exercise as a way to achieve ideal weight. A better way to appreciate the relationship between exercise and fat is to consider the fact that the energy you expend during a half hour of squash, handball, or raquetball played every day is equivalent to about nineteen pounds of fat per year—fat that otherwise would have accumulated in a year on the same diet without exercise.

In addition, your metabolic rate—the rate at which your body uses up energy or burns up calories—increases during exercise. Several studies indicate that your metabolic rate remains high for hours after your exercise session. One University of Southern California study reported that four hours after strenuous activity, the resting metabolic rate of the subjects was 7.5 percent to 28 percent higher than it would have been at the same time of day if they had not exercised. This fact alone would account for a yearly weight loss of four to five pounds.

Low back pain is a common problem in America. Recently, more than three hundred medical specialists met in Chicago to discuss this major health problem. It was disclosed that low back pain afflicts one in five adults and will cost our nation $81 million in 1987 alone.

According to reports, low back pain is the leading cause of worker disability, accounting for 25 percent of all claims. I see this firsthand. For many years I have set up health and fitness programs for all types of businesses. Most of the time I'm asked to incorporate a special program to prevent and alleviate low back pain, as it's the employees' number one complaint.

Most physicians agree that the major çause of low back pain is weak, out-of-shape abdominal muscles. When the abdominal muscles are weak, the pelvis tilts forward, which places an unusual strain on the discs of the spine. Pressure on the spinal discs can force fluid from the disc spaces. This puts pressure on the surrounding nerve roots, which is translated as pain, sometimes severe pain. Strong, fit abdominal muscles, which can be achieved through a consistent program of a variety of sit-ups, is a step in the right direction.

This list of exercise benefits would not be complete without noting that exercise is a way to increase your lifespan and help you look younger. Most people look much older than they should. When you see someone who looks young for his or her age, that is actually the way he or she should look.

In cultures around the world where living to one hundred years of age or more is common, exercise is always a natural and consistent part of the way of life. Even though many people from these cultures don't practice organized exercise as we know it—fitness centers, track clubs, and so on—they are physically active most of the time.

A recent study in the *New England Journal of Medicine* shows that regular exercise that burns 2000 calories or more per week can significantly reduce the risk of death. The research project, in which the mortality rate among 16,936 Harvard university graduates aged thirty-five to seventy-four was calculated over a sixteen-year period, produced some interesting findings: men who burned at least 2000 calories per week through exercise had a 28 percent lower death rate than less active men. And the death rate declined steadily as the energy expended during exercise increased from fewer than 500 calories to 3500 calories a week. But what's even more remarkable is that longevity was extended by exercise even when such health risk factors as smoking, high blood pressure, and obesity were present.

But a word of caution is in order. Even though you may be motivated to jump up right now and go exercise, it is advisable for you to first have a fitness checkup by your physician. This is especially important if you are age forty or older.

The benefits we've discussed so far—increased energy and sense of well-being, less tension, lower blood pressure, improved heart efficiency, freedom from constipation, freedom from circulation problems, and improved weight control—what they add up to is a person who is relaxed and energetic, vibrant and alive.

You can be that person! It's simply a matter of choice.

Yes, you can be that person if you are willing to take responsibility and consciously choose to achieve fitness. So you'll know what's involved in creating and maintaining the kind of fitness program that will result in positive changes for you, let me tell you about the three primary types of exercise.

The first exercise you should do before beginning any other fitness activities is stretching. During the course of a day, most people never stretch their calves, thighs, back, or arms, and, as a result, their bodies become rigid. Lack of movement, particularly along the spinal column, restricts nourishment to thousands of nerve endings, often results in lower back pain, and increases the chance of injury.

Stretching exercises are best performed just before and just after any vigorous exercise. As most professional fitness instructors will tell you, you should extend yourself to the point of stretch, not to the point of pain. My experience in working with others has been that, for those of you who haven't stretched in awhile, almost any stretching is painful. Your body simply isn't accustomed to the new position. It's not wise to ignore this fact and force yourself to bend farther than is comfortable by bouncing or yanking. Muscles and ligaments that are pulled too far will respond by contracting. Your short, tight muscles will become even shorter and tighter. Instead, pull yourself gently into the stretch and hold it for as long as you can, ideally for a minimum of sixty seconds. Then move on to another position. Because consistency and patience are the most important qualities you can bring to stretching, try to spend at least ten minutes each day working with your body.

Instead of sitting in a chair in front of the TV or sitting while reading, get into different stretch positions, preferably on the floor, so you can get two things done at once. You'll be amazed at how quickly your body will respond to this regular stretching and to the new demands. A generously illustrated book that covers everything you need to know about stretching is *Stretching*, by Bob Anderson.

I also recommend spending 5-30 minutes daily using some type of slant board. When you relax with your head lower than your feet, your entire body reaps the benefits. It's an easy, safe and effective means of allowing gravity to work for your body instead of against it. Everyday I use a slant board called BODYSLANT. This wonderful health product also functions as a lounge, bed and ottoman. The Bodyslant can help improve blood circulation to your brain, eyes, ears, gums, face and scalp. I also use the Bodyslant for visualization and meditation. (Refer to Resource Directory for more information.)

The second type of exercise involves strengthening and toning the muscles. Calisthenics will do this, but the best exercise in this category is weight lifting, or weight training. With a proper, effective weight training program you not only tone up, strengthen, and improve the definition of your muscles, but you also reshape your body. That's one of the wonderful things about weight training. you can actually zero in on any area of your body. For example, if you desire shapelier thighs or a flatter abdomen, you can work specifically on those areas. If you want tighter buttocks or larger pectorals, you can spend extra time on those areas.

Some women are reluctant to do weight training for fear they will develop large, defined muscles. For men, weight training will help develop muscle size as well as strength because the male hormone, testosterone, facilitates muscle fiber enlargement. A woman, however, lacking the same level of this hormone, cannot develop the muscle bulk her male counterpart can. It's that simple. Furthermore, a woman has larger, smoother muscle tissue and an extra layer of subcutaneous fat, which combine to soften body contours. Therefore, weight training can help reduce fatty tissue buildup while increasing strength and endurance, without a corresponding increase in muscle bulk.

Dumbells and hand, wrist, and ankle weights—which all fall into the category of free weights—can help build lean body tissue and muscle strength. The results of your workouts will be added definition and tone that help reproportion your body. Women will notice marked improvement, especially in the hips and buttocks, where fat tends to accumulate.

As your weight training regimen progresses, you'll be replacing fat with muscle mass. And though you may not notice a change on the scale, you'll be losing inches. Remember, people with well-conditioned muscles burn calories faster than those with extra fat. The reason is that muscle fiber demands more oxygen than fatty tissue does—and the more oxygen consumed, the more calories used as well. An excellent book to read on fitness is *Fit or Fat?* by Convert Bailey.

Free weights also allow explosive movements, letting you develop power more quickly than other exercises. In addition, they enable you to work on your performance in certain sports. For instance, concentrating on the buttocks muscles improves performance in gymnastics, ice skating, soccer, hockey, racquet sports, and basketball. Progressive weight training is also one of the best ways to strengthen the bones and to help prevent osteoporosis.

When you are working out with weights, whether free weights or machines, here are some key points to keep in mind. Always begin each exercise period with a warm-up and stretching routine. After you have stretched, do some brisk walking, do some jogging, or ride a bicycle for a few minutes in order to increase your heart rate and to warm your entire body. This is an excellent way to prevent injury and to get the most from your workout.

Never hold your breath when lifting weights. In fact, a complete inhalation and exhalation should take place with each repetition. You should inhale before exertion and exhale forcefully through the mouth during the lifting movement. (Example: During the leg press exercise, exhale as you approach full extension of the legs and inhale as you return to the beginning position.

All exercises should be performed with a full range of motion, that is, with full extension and contraction of the muscles involved. No matter how heavy the resistance, you should concentrate on making your muscles contract deliberately through their entire range of motion. This stimulates the natural resistance phenomenon of most athletic movements. Also, an intense, all-out effort is necessary to gain the maximum training benefit. Weights should be returned to the starting position in a controlled manner.

You should also develop a fast, steady pace with almost no pause between repetitions. Train to move from one station to the next with a minimum of rest. If you have to wait for someone ahead of you to finish, jog in place or skip rope to maintain your target heart rate (to be explained later). This way you will also be improving your endurance.

To build more strength and bulk, do fewer repetitions with more weight; to tone and streamline, increase the number of repetitions and reduce the amount of weight. Ideally, beginners should train for thirty to forty-five minutes three or four times a week, with at least one full day of rest between sessions.

Wear loose-fitting clothes so you will not restrict movement, plus athletic shoes with cushiony soles and plenty of support.

When lifting, keep your abdominals tight, to avoid overstressing your back. Further, keep your wrists straight. This not only prevents injury, but also makes the workout more effective.

After a workout you should not head for the showers until your pulse rate, breathing and perspiration have returned to a normal resting state. Gradually decrease body movement in the same way you progressively warmed it up prior to the exercise session. This keeps the blood circulating, helps prevent dizziness, and lets your system unwind.

To reap the most from your workouts, you'll want to work out three times a week, even if you are an advanced lifter. Another option is four, five, or six times a week, alternating body parts so that each body part that's been worked out has a full day's rest before the next training session. If you also cycle or jog, you could jog on the days that you don't lift, or maybe use your jog as the warm-up before you lift. What's most important is that you create

a program that fits well into your way of life so you will welcome
it rather than resist it.

I regularly go to a gym for my weight training. At home, I also
have, and highly recommend, a few pieces of equipment to supplement the gym and to use when I can't get away to the weight room.
I have set up several home and office minifitness centers for clients,
and there's really a lot you can do with a limited space and a little
ingenuity. I recommend starting with a basic bench along with
some pairs of dumbbells, and perhaps some barbells. If your
budget allows, you may want to consider one of the compact mul-
tistation machines. For information on home or office exercise
equipment, or if you want to receive a poster/chart I developed that
is entitled "Over 100 Ways Exercise Will Enrich the Quality of Your
Life," please write to Universal Gym Equipment, Inc.; the address
is listed in the resource directory.

In regard to calisthenics, I have some advice regarding sit-ups.
Lower back problems can be helped by strengthening and toning
the abdominal muscles. Consider spending a few minutes each day
on this area. Here's a training tip to hasten results for intermediate
and advanced fitness enthusiasts. Rather than doing one hundred
to two hundred sit-ups in a row, you'll get more benefit from doing
fewer of them with increased resistance. The way to increase resistance when you're doing sit-ups is to use a slant board or to hold
a weight behind your neck. My weight training partner, Jesse
Castañeda, and I do a variety of sit-ups, always using weights to
add that extra resistance for better results.

The third type of exercise is endurance-type aerobic activity, or
cardio-vascular conditioning. It is aerobic exercise that affects your
heart rate, blood vessels, and lung capacity. Aerobic exercise will
probably do more for you than any other form of exercise to
increase your life span.

Did you know that when the body is at rest the human heart
beats an average of 72 times a minute, 4300 times an hour, 104,000
times a day—2.8 billion times in a lifetime of 74 years? But no heart
is at its resting pace for a lifetime. It speeds up with exertion, be it
exercising, love making, or grocery shopping. What a wonderful
thing you do for your heart when you engage in regular, vigorous

cardiovascular exercise! This type of exercise makes the heart a more efficient pump and lowers the resting heart rate. Thus, your fit heart will pump the same amount of blood (or perhaps slightly more) as the nonfit heart of another, and it won't have to work as hard. Through regular, vigorous cardiovascular exercise you give your heart the gift of lifetime efficiency.

Some of the more popular aerobic exercises are:

Fitness Walking (also known as striding)   This is one of the best, most underrated of all exercises. Walking exercises the entire body in a gentle but consistent manner. Walking involves little risk of overstressing the cardiovascular or the musculoskeletal system. It is an exercise that can be enjoyed by almost everyone, even far into old age. For full benefit, walking must be done with a purposeful, full-strided, brisk gait, arms swinging vigorously.

Fitness walking just may be the perfect exercise for the person who hates to exercise. It requires no special skill or equipment; a comfortable pair of good walking shoes is all you need. The walking shoes (and aerobic, hiking, tennis and jogging shoes) I wear are the New Balance brand. You can lose weight and tone and strengthen your entire body. If it's cardiovascular fitness you're after, striding at a brisk pace for a sufficient amount of time will give your heart a workout that's almost the equivalent of a vigorous run—without the risk of injuries.

Here are some pointers to remember about fitness walking. A full arm swing is important for balance and rhythm. It helps tone your upper body and gives you the momentum you need, especially when walking on an incline. Correct posture is also important. Stand tall, with your chin held high, back straight, and stomach and buttocks tucked in. Your head and torso should be aligned with your lower body; leaning forward can cause fatigue and back pain. Finally, you will walk faster and run the risk of fewer injuries if you place your feet properly. Your toes should point forward. Place the outside of your heel firmly on the ground, then roll forward toward the ball of your foot, raising your heel. This procedure is necessary to avoid landing flat-footed. Next, push off the ball of your foot and toes, placing one foot in front of the other not more than a few inches apart (otherwise your body will sway unnecessarily). For more information on this, you may refer to any book on fitness walking.

> The sovereign invigorator of the body is exercise, and of all the exercises walking is the best.
> —Thomas Jefferson

Jogging This is one step above walking in terms of pace and benefits, but also in potential risks. It involves more efficient stimulation of circulation and respiration, and thus gives better immediate and long-term benefits. It can, however, place added stress on the feet, knees, and hips, and that can sometimes lead to injury.

Running This is next on the ladder and is only for a small percentage of people. Unless you are of a lighter and slighter build, running may not be for you. (The exception is shorter periods of running during interval training, that is, short bouts of running during your jogging session or the alternating of days of running and days of jogging.) The risk of injury in running is proportionally greater than in jogging or brisk walking. There is also the excitement and satisfaction of competition. Not all races are marathons, of course, and even the jogger may find an occasional five-kilometer or ten-kilometer (6.2 miles) race interesting and stimulating.

Try to walk, jog, or run on soft, natural surfaces, especially if you are just beginning an exercise program. Be sure to wear a good pair of shoes. This is the most important consideration, so carefully select the best shoe for your feet.

Swimming This is a terrific exercise because it allows for aerobic exertion and improved flexibility, with very little stress on muscles or bones—unless you run into a big fish, which actually has happened to me! I prefer ocean-swimming to swimming in a pool, and do so on a regular basis. If you swim in a pool, I recommend that you wear a good pair of goggles and always rinse off when you have finished, so the chlorinated water won't dry out your skin and hair.

Aerobic Dance Lots of people gravitate toward this type of exercise because of group motivation and social ambience. Aerobic dance, if done properly, can improve lung capacity, muscle flexibilty, and strength. Sessions that are conducted too fast or with severe, jarring movements, however, can lead to muscle and joint problems. Start off slowly and always wear good, supportive shoes.

Bicycling—Here is one of my favorite exercises. It is less jarring than jogging or running, and can be easily adapted to the beginning or the advanced exerciser. It affords the opportunity to exercise alone or with others and to see many different sights. For those of you who get bored easily, cycling might be just right for you. By the way, don't forget the stationary bicycle. It's excellent if you live in a densely populated area or in a climate that makes it difficult to exercise outdoors. Choose one with a tension gauge, so you can adjust it to meet your appropriate exercising heart rate.

It is important to incorporate cross-training into your exercise program. This helps to relieve boredom, keep you motivated and ensure that all your different muscle groups will be exercised. Outdoors, I enjoy ocean-swimming, jogging, walking and cycling. Indoors, I workout on my PRECOR fitness equipment. I have a climber, treadmill, stationary bicycle, and rower. This combination works well for me. Each day I participate in a different aerobic activity. For example, my weekly routine might look like this: Monday – climber; Tuesday – jobbing; Wednesday – rower; Thursday – cycling; Friday – treadmill; Saturday – walking; Sunday – stationary bicycle.

Other aerobic activities include cross-country skiing, rebounding (on a minitrampoline), jumping rope, and roller skating.

To achieve best results with aerobic activity, you must increase your heart rate to a minimum level and keep it at that rate for thirty minutes, at least three times a week. (Six times a week for twenty minutes will produce similar results.) Naturally, if you haven't exercised in quite a while, you'll need to build up to that level slowly. For example, if you've selected jogging as your endurance activity, you will start off by walking, then walking and slow jogging, then all slow jogging until finally you're able to jog the entire thirty minutes without stopping or being completely winded. This might take four weeks or longer if you are a beginner.

You can monitor your present level of fitness and your improvement by keeping track of your heart rate. Basically, the slower your resting heart rate, the higher your level of fitness. Your resting heart rate is the rate at which your heart beats when you are not physically active, such as just before you get up in the morning. For most people the resting heart rate is between seventy and eighty beats per minute. These averages are derived from insurance surveys that include unfit, overweight people. Many athletes have resting heart rates of fifty beats per minute, and some have resting heart rates as low as forty. That means an athlete's heart might be working only half as hard as that of most sedentary individuals to pump the same amount of blood.

To determine your own heart rate, place your index and middle fingers (not your thumb) on one of two places on the body: the carotid arteries, running along both sides of the front of the neck, or the radial arteries, located on the inside of the forearm, the thumb side of the wrist. Other places where the pulse can be measured are the inner thigh, the navel region, and the sides of the head near the eyes. (You've probably felt this pulse without even trying when you've had a headache.)

To get an accurate picture of your resting heart rate, take your pulse every morning for a week. Place your finger on one of the pulse points and count the beats for fifteen seconds. Multiply the number of beats by four to get your resting heart rate per minute. Be sure to take your pulse as soon as you awake in the morning, while you are still in bed, because many factors can stimulate your heartbeat, such as foods, caffeine, tobacco, coughing, or even talking. Once you've determined your resting heart rate, you have a means of measuring your progress.

As you strengthen your body's cardiovascular system—heart, vessels, and lungs—you will lower your resting heart rate, and a decreased resting heart rate means your heart has become a more efficient organ. It doesn't have to beat as often to pump the same amount of blood.

If, like the motor in your car, which has a life span of miles, your heart has a life span of beats, you can add years to your life by slowing down the beating of your heart. (An added benefit of regular exercise is that you'll still be in good condition, so you can enjoy those added years.)

The best way yet discovered to lower your resting heart rate is, paradoxically, to make it beat faster during periods of exercise. That's what aerobic exercise does. *Aerobic* means "with oxygen," although at the beginning of your aerobics program you'll probably feel as though you're "without oxygen." As I said earlier, the purpose of aerobic exercise is to increase endurance, and to accomplish this you must place enough stress on your heart to substantially increase your heart rate. (See chart on page 225.)

You will want to exercise with your heart rate in a certain target training zone to reap the most benefits. your approximate target exercising heart rate can be established with this formula:

(220 – your age) × 60% (conservative target exercising heart rate for the beginner) Example: 220 – 40 years old or 180 × 60% = 108 target heart rate

(220 – your age) × 70-75% (intermediate target exercising heart rate)

(220 – your age) × 80-85% (advanced target exercising heart rate)

The way you monitor your heart rate during exercise is to count your pulse for six seconds and multiply it by ten to get your active pulse rate per minute. Because your heart rate will slow down immediately when you stop exercising, try to take your pulse during the activity or immediately upon stopping.

Let's assume, as an example, that at the age of forty, you have taken up jogging as your aerobic exercise. You've been jogging about ten minutes one day when you decide to check your pulse. It registers 90 beats per minute. You know that your resting heart rate is 70 beats per minute. To get the full aerobic benefit, you must get your exercise heart rate up to between 108 and 126 beats per minute, so pick up the pace a little. If you are an advanced jogger at age forty, your exercise heart rate needs to be approximately 144-153 beats per minute (220 – 40 × 80-85%).

Now if it sounds as though you will turn into a fanatical pulse-taker, you needn't worry. After awhile, you will tune into your body well enough to know what your pulse is without actually taking it. You'll be able to tell from your breathing, perspiration rate, and ability to talk while jogging.

Another good indication of your level of fitness is the speed with which your pulse drops to normal after exercise. Just as you are finishing your exercises, take your pulse. Then wait one minute and take your pulse again. It should drop at least ten beats per minute during that time. After twenty minutes your pulse should be much closer to your normal "moving around" heart rate. The better conditioned you become, the more quickly your heart rate will drop to normal after exercise.

When beginning an exercise program, keep in mind the following points:

1. *Select exercises and activities you find enjoyable. For example, if you love the outdoors and enjoy visiting different places, why not take up cycling as your aerobic activity. Or try a combination of brisk walking, cycling, and roller skating.*

2. *Train, don't strain, especially if you're just beginning to work out after a long layoff. It has probably taken several years to get your body in the shape it's in today, so don't expect to reverse the process in two weeks.*

3. *Reward and pamper yourself for your efforts. Soak in the tub or jacuzzi, have a massage, enjoy a sauna—but whatever you do, don't give up. Repetition is the key to mastery in every area of your life.*

As I said earlier, it takes at least twenty-one days for your mind and body to create a new habit. Until then, you can expect to have to listen to that incessant voice in the back of your mind. I call that voice Babbler. You can count on Babbler to keep up a running monologue on how nice it would be to sleep late, how sore your calf muscles are, or how heavy the weights feel. Babbler will probably tell you that you look just fine the way you are, that people who really love you don't care about a few extra pounds or inches, or that huffing and puffing at the top of the stairs is normal for someone of your age.

Don't pay any attention. Instead, when the commentary begins, simply acknowledge Babbler's point of view, let it go, and then remind yourself that for twenty-one days you are going to stick to your new exercise program. If at the end of that time you feel you aren't benefitting from it, you can reevaluate. By the end of twenty-one days, chances are you'll no longer have any resistance to exercising. In fact, it's likely you'll have become positively addicted to it.

I am often asked about spot reducing—is it possible and how can one make it work quickly? I'm sorry to tell you that trying to spot reduce is futile, although you can spot condition and spot firm through weight training.

A recent study, conducted by Frank Katch, Ed.D., and his associates at the University of Massachusetts, looked at the effects of spot exercising on subjects who performed 5000 sit-ups over twenty-seven days. The subjects' abdominal muscles became stronger and more well-defined, and they also showed a decrease in fat on the abdomens, backs, and buttocks—even though this exercise works primarily the abdominal muscles. The study did, however, rule out the possibility that spot reducing could be effective.

It's important to realize that although exercise doesn't work as a spot reducer, it can form and strengthen weak and flabby musculature. Many people have protruding abdomens not because they are excessively fat, but because their weak muscles allow the abdominal organs to push against the abdominal wall, which then protrudes. Sit-ups, reverse sit-ups, and curl-ups are effective in firming this area and producing an attractively strong and slim abdomen.

Why you lose fat and *where* is something researchers are still debating. Some feel that you lose mostly from those areas that have the most fat. Others feel that fat comes off the area where it was most recently deposited. Genetics probably has a lot to do with where you'll lose.

In regard to fitness in the work world, there is a rapidly growing trend toward establishing in-house health and fitness facilities. In my consulting, I have seen how fitness programs improve employee morale and help decrease illness and therefore use of sick-leave and insurance claims. All this adds up to increased sales and productivity. My experience shows me that companies can't afford not to provide some type of fitness program for their staff.

Finally, three more elements can make your fitness program, and hence your life, a great adventure. Goals, visualizations, and affirmations are all important elements to staying motivated to exercise.

It is essential to set goals. If you don't have a goal, you won't have much incentive to stick with your program. Goals provide a path, a direction, and let you know how you are doing. What are your goals for exercising? To lose weight and reshape your body? To increase your energy and boost your self-esteem? Perhaps you want to be able to run in a 10K race or increase your strength and muscle definition. Whatever is important to you, write it down. Keep in mind that just because goals are on paper doesn't mean they can't be modified later. Really give thought to what you want to achieve in your exercise program.

Goals are both short-term and long-term. This means that you can make, for example, three lists of goals—one for the next month, one for the next six months, and one for the entire year. Be realistic; don't set yourself up to fail. If you've just started a jogging program and can now go one mile nonstop, don't make one of your goals to be able to run a marathon at the end of the month. I'm not saying that it's impossible, but it is unlikely.

After you've written your list, post it where you can see it every day, perhaps on the refrigerator door or on the bathroom mirror. As you achieve your goals, rewrite them. In addition to a concise list of goals, make another list of your plans for achieving your goals. Let's say that you've been jogging for six months and you're now up to three miles, three times a week. Your goals might be to run a 10K in six months, a marathon after that, and to increase your strength and lose inches by lifting weights. You'd then map out a jogging program that gradually increases your mileage weekly, in addition to working on a specific weight training program to suit your needs. This is the procedure I followed when training to run 100 miles, from Santa Barbara to Los Angeles.

It's a good idea to read your goals daily and to evaluate your progress weekly, to make sure you're staying on course.

I have always found it beneficial to confide in caring friends and tell them my goals. Oftentimes it's easy to let yourself down and break commitments, but it's harder to get off the course when a supportive friend is checking up to see how you're progressing. Make sure it's a trusted friend with whom you feel comfortable and not someone who will bring up your "slip-ups" or "goofs" whenever you get together.

You must also control your thinking. Think only positive, encouraging, uplifting thoughts. Let go of all fearful or doubting thoughts. Think of all the reasons why you can succeed. Of course, this goes for all areas of your life, not just your fitness goals.

So *watch your thoughts!* As I discussed earlier, every one of us is the sum total of his or her thoughts. We are where we are because that is exactly where we want to be, whether we realize it or not.

You must also act the part of the fit and healthy person you have decided to become. In other words, act as though it were impossible to fail. Be fit and healthy, aligning with that desire in everything you think, feel, say, and do.

When you are clear on the fitness goal you want to achieve and you've written it down, make sure you expect the best. In *The Power of Positive Thinking,* Norman Vincent Peale says that "when you expect the best, you release a magnetic force in your mind which by law of attraction tends to bring the best to you."

Finally, the success of your exercise program is greatly influenced by your attitude toward that program. Stay enthusiastic about your goals. "Nothing great was ever achieved without enthusiasm," said Emerson. With a positive attitude toward achieving your fitness goals, it will be easier to persist in the right direction. By being persistent, you are demonstrating faith. Persistence is simply another word for faith; if you didn't have faith, you'd never persist.

Remember that your subconscious stores all of your thoughts and experiences in the same way that a computer stores the data it is fed. If your thoughts are primarily negative, your subconscious computer attempts to create experiences that are in alignment with your negative viewpoint. On the other hand, if you see your exercise program as a challenge rather than a burden, and fully expect that you will complete your exercise goals, your subconscious will assist in creating that reality.

As before, let's assume that jogging is your aerobic activity. What are your beliefs about yourself as a jogger? Do you compare yourself to other joggers and judge yourself inadequate? Do you set up impossible jogging goals for yourself and then feel guilty when you don't meet them? Do you frequently make agreements with yourself to jog in the morning and then oversleep instead? If you answered yes to any of these questions, be aware that you are negatively programming your jogging plans. Each time you create expectations of yourself that you don't meet, you lower your self-esteem. And that creates even more negativity, because you begin to doubt yourself and your ability to keep agreements.

The best way to break that cycle is through positive visualizations and affirmations. Twice a day, just as you wake up in the morning and just as you fall asleep at night, create a positive fantasy, a mental movie that supports your new exercise program. Engage your imagination to create a vivid fantasy in which you see yourself keeping your agreements and achieving your goals. For example, if you usually jog early in the morning, create a wonderful fantasy of rising early, feeling completely rested and awake. When you begin your stretching, you are amazed at how flexible your body is feeling today. In your mind see exactly how far you are able to stretch, and feel your satisfaction in your progress. Now imagine yourself stepping outside. The weather is perfect. The morning is quiet except for the sound of the singing birds, and a gentle, soothing breeze lifts your hair and softly brushes against your face. If you usually jog with someone else, include him or her in your mental movie. Imagine that you are beginning your jog. Your legs feel strong, you have good balance, and your feet are striking the ground squarely. An incredible surge of energy and well-being permeates your body, and you are very glad to be out jogging. Based on your level of training, you have set a reasonable, but challenging, mileage goal for yourself. Imagine yourself nearing the end of the run, feeling like you could actually run much farther. If you jog the same course each day, see yourself reaching the end of the course and feel the elation of a great workout. Your skin is radiant, your body feels purified, and your mind is totally alert. Allow yourself to experience that moment for awhile, and then see yourself returning home and going about your daily routine feeling very pleased with yourself.

That's one example of how to set up a mental movie. Here are the key points to remember in creating your fitness mental movie. Phrase all suggestions positively, such as, "I am able to jog farther and faster today than ever before." If you make the suggestion in the negative, such as, "When I jog today I will not get a sideache," your subconscious mind may hear, "When I jog today I will get a sideache." Another key point is to make sure that all your suggestions are present tense. Tell yourself, "Every day in every way I am becoming a better jogger," rather then "By the end of July, I will be able to jog three miles a day." The subconscious has no conception of time, so suggestions for the future will remain just that, in the future.

The final point, and by far the most important, is to become totally involved in your movie. Use every ounce of your imagination to create a movie that is real: perceive it clearly in your mind, imagine conversations and feel the positive emotions. All of these things will make the movie many times more powerful than if you perceived it as a casual observer.

Of course this is not to say that through visualization and affirmation alone you can achieve your fitness goals without ever having to work out physically. Not at all! But integrating these techniques into your exercise program will enrich your adventure and hasten achievement of all your fitness goals. Keep in mind, repetition is the key to mastery. And stay disciplined. Discipline is the ability to carry out your resolutions long after the mood has left you.

Actress Linda Evans of television's "Dynasty" exemplifies the importance and benefits of incorporating the principles shared in this book. She follows a sound diet and gets plenty of exercise, but the real secret, she says, is visualization. Evans takes the "You are what you eat" adage one step further, adding that "You are what you think." She recently explained her philosophy to a U.S. Senate panel on nutrition and fitness: "Like countless American men and women," she said, "I want to be the best 'me' I can be—and I believe fitness plays a vital role in achieving that goal. As a woman in my forties, I have learned that I am capable of changing what I don't like about my life. You don't have to fall apart because you are getting older. However, if you believe that you'll begin to fall apart in your thirties, you probably will."

Evans lifts weights and jogs regularly. She also says that before starting any new diet, she first visualizes how she eventually wants to look, which helps keep her motivated.

"It's never too late," she says, "to change our views and adjust our thinking. All of us who want to improve ourselves can do so. It just takes work."

And to do the work, of course, takes motivation. Take notice when you are not as motivated to work out. What's going on in your life? Does your exercise program lack variety? Is the program an emotional challenge? Are you pushing too hard? Have you decided that getting in shape is not a top priority for you? Keep in mind that you are working out for yourself, not to please someone else. Others can provide an incentive, but the prime reason must come from your own desire.

So don't put it off any longer. Choose today to make fitness a top priority. Exercise or lack thereof, does indeed affect the body. And whatever affects the body positively also has a positive effect on the mind, as well as enriching awareness of the Spirit within. Similarly, lack of exercise, which brings physical deterioration, has a negative effect on the mind. Those of us who exercise regularly know what I mean; those who don't have yet to discover feeling radiantly alive.

Keeping this holistic approach in mind—and in body and spirit—we can see how exercise will do wonders to enhance well-being. You owe it to yourself to take the best care of your body that you can, and you need to recognize and acknowledge the benefits you're accruing from your fitness program. You are meant to be healthy, vibrantly alive, radiantly fit. But to be healthy just for the sake of being healthy is, I believe, missing the mark. Our bodies are the beautiful temples for the Spirit that lives within every one of us. The more you care for yourself and do those things that bring about greater health and well-being, the more you are able to get in touch with your real Self—that shining center of love and light within.

Be continually thankful for your miraculous body and all its wondrous functions. Thank your body and God by taking good care of yourself. The better you take care of yourself, the easier it will be to live fully, to live in balance, and to be filled with vibrant health. It is up to you. No one is going to exercise for you. You must take responsibility for your own health. Make a commitment, today. Stay disciplined. Choose to be fit and healthy. If you do, I guarantee that you will not only look better, but you will feel better, think more clearly, and have a more positive attitude about yourself and life.

Self-Discovery Questions

1. *What is my resting heart rate and my target exercising heart rate?*

2. *How do I feel about exercise?*

3. *What beliefs do I have about my exercise that have been working against me?*

4. *What excuses seem to frequently come up that interfere with my exercising?*

5. *Here are my exercise and fitness goals for the following month, three months, six months, and year.*

6. *The areas of my body that need special attention are:*

7. *My body is miraculous. Here are a few of the numerous body functions for which I am grateful:*

Action Choices

1. For the next twenty-one days I will do the following exercises:

2. Here is an outline of my fitness goals for the next twenty-one days:

3. Among the things I can change about my body, I choose to change the following, by using this outlined approach:

4. After twenty-one days of consistently exercising, here are some of my thoughts and feelings about exercise, my program, my body, and myself.

5. *Listed here are at least two physical activities I've wanted to try but have not yet begun.*

6. *Listed here are ways I can increase my everyday physical activity. (For example, I can carry my own grocery bags, or I can park a few blocks away from my destination and walk briskly the rest of the way.)*

7. *Because my _____ needs extra attention to improve fitness, for twenty-one consistent days I will exercise it specifically by doing the following exercises:*

CHOOSE TO

BE MORE CHILDLIKE

This ability to see, experience and accept the new is one of our saving characteristics. To be fearful of tomorrow, to close ourselves to possibilities, to resist the inevitable, to advocate standing still when all else is moving forward, is to lose touch. If we accept the new with joy and wonder, we can move gracefully into each tomorrow. More often than not, the children shall lead us.

—Leo Buscaglia, Bus 9 to Paradise

So many people are searching for the fountain of youth, the secret that will enable them to live a long and full life. Some follow strict diets, exercise vigorously, or swear by expensive supplements. Yet few have looked deeply enough to understand that the secret to living a life full of aliveness and fulfillment lies within. And this secret is expressed in our attitude, our expression, our thoughts, and how we view ourselves and the world around us. Forever my inspiration and teachers, young children have much to teach us about experiencing life to the fullest.

A couple of years ago I decided to have a party to which I invited several neighborhood children. The party took place in my backyard. The children ranged in age from three to six. Just before the party began I received an upsetting telephone call. The caller was a close friend and we were not seeing eye to eye on something important to both of us. We started out calmly but ended up with higher blood pressures, raised voices, and feelings of frustration.

I went back outside to greet my young guests as they arrived. The toys were ready, the decorations were ready, the snacks were ready—and I was ready to call the whole thing off. I'm so glad I didn't. That day became one of the most significant days of my life. Within no time at all, I forgot about my telephone conversation and got involved with the children, allowing myself to become a child again.

As time went by I began to realize that children instinctively understand the secret of living fully. Their moments appear to be almost magical as they are totally fascinated by their world, unmindful of the problems of yesterday or tomorrow. Somehow children are able to let go and embrace life with passion. They are able to give themselves permission to be free, to be totally absorbed in the present, and to embrace the unfamiliar and the out of the ordinary.

How often do you do this? When was the last time you tried something different, something totally unusual? It can add tremendous adventure and fulfillment to your life. As you move out of your usual sphere, the boundaries of your reality expand and your experience of aliveness deepens. It may be something as simple as trying a new foreign food or taking a different route to work. Or it could be taking your family to an unfamiliar place one weekend.

I thrive in embracing the unfamiliar, although it hasn't always been this way for me. For example, in the Summer of 1986, I was invited to speak on Wellness at John Denver's first annual symposium, "Choices for the Future," in Snowmass, Colorado. My usual plan would be to fly in, participate in the festivities, and then fly home or on to another destination. Instead, I decided to drive alone several days ahead of schedule with the goal of just being, enjoying the scenery, taking pictures, stopping when I felt like it—all the while keeping my full attention in the present moment. This solitary experience filled me with tremendous joy and peace. Upon arriving in Snowmass I was given a beautiful condominium to stay in while I was there, but I decided that first night to do something different: I decided to sleep outside alone in the mountains of Colorado. So, with some uncertainty, before dark I hiked high up a mountain with a willingness to enjoy this special time. It turned out to be one of the most inspiring nights of my life, as I embraced the stars, the animals, the insects, the cold, and the energy of the night. And it's the children who have taught me best to give myself permission to try new things, to expand my experience of life.

I have always had a great fondness for children. While I was still living with my family, during high school and my first year at UCLA, the children of the neighborhood would often come to my home to see if I could come out and play. I could rarely resist. And I can remember with great vividness the games we would play, the hours we laughed, the endless moments when we were silly and goofy. Those times will always hold a special place in my heart. When was the last time you played hide-and-go-seek with some children, or tag, or pin the tail on the bush? I recall with warmth the hours I spent as a child riding my bike, pretending it was a magnificent white stallion, and as I rode, the horse and I were like one, galloping strongly and swiftly, the wind gently embracing my face and hair.

Even today some of my best times are had with children. Each year I take a group of children to Disneyland or the circus, and I can often be found at my local park, playground, or beach with some small friends, playing ball, swinging, running, feeding birds, or just laughing a lot.

I can also remember the numerous times during my life that adults have asked me why I didn't act my age. I figure that as long as I continue to hear that, I must be doing just fine.

My greatest adult teacher in showing me the value and joy of being childlike has been Wayne Dyer. Prolific author and producer of audiocassettes, he is a shining example of the magic blending of both adult and child. In his book *What Do You Really Want for Your Children*, he shares his thoughts about his love for children and how important it has been for him to let his childlike quality shine forth. The first time I met Wayne, he was wearing his Mickey Mouse tee-shirt and he had that spark of aliveness and joyfulness so apparent in young children.

I am reminded of something I heard Buckminster Fuller once say. "I have great hope for tomorrow. And my hope lies in the following three things: truth, youth, and love."

There is a distinct difference between being childlike and being childish. To be childish means either to be a child and act like one, which is perfectly normal, or to be an adult and act like a child in ways that indicate your growth and maturity were somehow impeded and you have been stagnating ever since.

To be childlike means to be innocent of strange, authoritarian ideas of what adulthood ought to be; to be trusting and straightforward; and to be more concerned with your experience of life than how you look to others.

It is important to understand that you do not have to give up being an adult in order to become more childlike. You do not have to become infantile or in the least bit irresponsible or unaccountable. The fully integrated person incorporates a harmonious blending of adult and child.

Within each of us is a child waiting to come forth and express itself more fully. What usually keeps us from getting back in touch with the child within is our own unwillingness to recognize and accept that child. It seems we often feel that "now that I'm grown up, I have to act my age." There is a lovely passage in the Bible, Matthew 19:14, that says, "Let the children come to me, and do not hinder them; for to such belongs the kingdom of heaven." Yes, young children live in their own heaven, no matter what their background, what language they speak, or where they live. Their celebration of life, their passion and joy is universal. I see this wherever I travel. Not too long ago, while jogging in a park in Switzerland, I noticed several children playing a game that was new to me. Their parents and guardians were sitting quietly, not talking to each other or paying much attention to the children. The kids were having a fantastic time—laughing, running, touching, being silly—just enjoying each other's company. It looked like so much fun. After watching for a few minutes, I felt compelled to join them. Through hand signals I asked if I could play. An hour later I was exhausted. Although I could not speak their language, there was still a special bonding and love, a respect and sharing that transcended the need for words. Laughing can be so freeing and so uniting at the same time.

The following day, toward the end of my walk, I noticed a little boy and little girl both down on all fours, looking keenly at the ground next to a beautiful flowering violet tree. I stopped to see what was so captivating. In broken English their mother told me that for nearly thirty minutes the two children had been engrossed in watching the movement of some ants as they made their journey from a tree to some bread crumbs a few feet away. At that moment I got down on my hands and knees and for several precious minutes I joined the children in their adventure, letting myself get totally involved with them and the ants. It was wonderfully delightful.

The children at my party all had something in common that transcended words—the joy of living fully, of celebrating life and each moment. Part of living fully is laughing a lot. This means laughing not only at the everyday incongruities of life but most especially at ourselves, as children do so well.

It's fun to be around people who can let their inner child come out to play. These are usually happy, fully functioning people who have not forgotten that it is possible to be happy and responsible at the same time; who aren't afraid of what others think; who can occasionally become totally immersed in fantasy, just as they did when they were children.

Take advantage of the many opportunities you have to let your inner child out for a great adventure. I sometimes get my friends involved. For example, I love the Jim Henson Muppet productions on TV and at the movies. Recently one of the Muppet specials was on TV. To celebrate this fun-filled adventure fantasy with Kermit the Frog and his companions, I invited over a few close friends to watch this show with me. I made two requests. The first, to come dressed as a little child, and the second, to bring a favorite toy. My very special teddy bear, Golden, and I greeted the guests. Ah! To let your inner child out to play is such a glorious gift—free and available to all.

I am reminded of a beautiful friend, Molly, who was all of 4'10" tall, but a giant of a woman. Well into her seventies when I met her, she knew how to let her inner child come out. The times we spent visiting together will always be special to me. A vibrant, alive, positive woman, Molly spent her days swimming, walking, doing yoga, or volunteering at the UCLA hospital.

About six months before she died, she found out she had cancer. The shocking news darkened her sunny attitude for the first three days. Then she adjusted to it and decided to make the most of her remaining days. She continued her routine, and seemed as radiantly alive and cheerful as ever.

The last month of her life she spent in the hospital. I was away on a lengthy tour, and when I returned I immediately visited Molly in the hospital. I wasn't prepared for what I saw. During my absence she had lost nearly half her body weight, all her teeth, most of her color, but astonishingly, not her cheerful attitude. Although she was physically unrecognizable, her spirit shone through when she said, "Sunny, I know I've looked better. Let's see if you can perform your magic and fix me up." I asked the nurse to leave Molly and me alone for awhile. I dropped the sidebars on her bed, and we celebrated being together. I brushed her hair, washed her face, and applied a drop of her favorite perfume. Although she could barely move, and she had a difficult time speaking, she still told me a couple of jokes. She also spoke with great appreciation about the flowers in her room and the birds singing to her from the tree outside her window. She then asked me to lie down next to her, because she needed to talk and she didn't think she had much time left. That final hour she spoke to me about the light and colors she saw and about the peaceful and joyful feeling she felt. Just before she died she said to me, "Life is meant to be joyful. Don't ever get too serious about life. Laugh every day and live each day as though it were your last. Every day let your inner child out to play. Always follow your heart and let the beauty of life into your spirit." And then she passed on.

Molly reminded me that we must embrace all of life and live every day as though we were born anew. Erich Fromm said, "Living is the process of continuous rebirth. The tragedy in the life of most of us is that we die before we are fully born." My experiences with Molly also make me think of something Elisabeth Kubler-Ross said in her book *Death: The Final Stage of Growth*.

> What is important is to realize that whether we understand fully who we are or what will happen when we die, it's our purpose to grow as human beings, to look within ourselves, to find and build upon that source of peace and understanding and strength that is our individual self. And then to reach out to others with love and acceptance and patient guidance in the hope of what we may become together.

This is what Molly did with me.

And then there was Isabelle. I met her when she was ninety-three, the last year of her life. We were both at a photocopy store, where she was making copies of her latest poetry manuscript. I overheard her asking for a telephone to call a taxi. So I introduced myself and offered to take her home. You can imagine my surprise when I found out she lived three doors away from me, having recently moved in. I'll always treasure the year I spent getting to know Isabelle. She showed me the insignificance of chronological age. Young in spirit, Isabelle loved to laugh, most especially at herself. She valued life's simple beauty—clouds, flowers, leaves, rain.

She loved to take a "blind trust walk" with me. Either in our homes, at the beach or at the park, we would walk arm in arm. One of us would have our eyes closed as we walked and explored together. When I was the blind partner she would lead me around for about fifteen minutes, introducing me to all kinds of sensory experiences—the sound of birds or waves, the smell of herbs, the touch of leaves or flowers. It's a fantastic way to practice living in the moment, to heighten awareness, and to learn about trust, letting go and embracing the unfamiliar.

A few weeks before her death, we were visiting, drinking tea and sharing ideas on world peace. Unexpectedly, it started to rain and Isabelle decided we should take off our shoes and walk outside and celebrate the rain and wet grass. I wish you could have seen her. Ageless and shining, she frolicked barefoot on the freshly cut grass, laughing, singing, and catching raindrops in her mouth. Yes, Isabelle, my precious friend, knew how to let her child out to play.

Clearly Molly and Isabelle knew that real life was not all work and no play. In fact, they made their work their play. They retained a childlike innocence and curiosity about being alive. Although they knew how to be an adult, they allowed their child within to be integrated into their days. Do you know people like this? If so, compare how you feel when you are around them with being around people who have not gotten in touch with their inner child. Menius, an ancient Greek philosopher, said, "The great man is he who does not lose his child's heart."

Now reflect a moment on your own experiences being around children. What are the children like? How do you feel when you are with them? What qualities do they express to you? Before you read on, write down what comes to mind when you think about children.

Study your list for a moment. How many of these qualities are part of your personality? Which ones would you like to develop or reawaken?

When I wrote my list, that evening after my neighborhood party, here is what I came up with: Children are cheerful, alert, eager, trusting, persevering, and open. They are also energetic, caring, sensitive, friendly, and inquisitive. They are enthusiastic, playful, expressive, spontaneous, and natural. They laugh a lot and love to act silly and crazy. They are also incredibly lovable and innocently loving. From my perspective, these natural childlike qualities are the true essence of living fully.

As children grow older they are strongly influenced by the mores and behavioral patterns of their role models and their society. It is a shame to see that the models of adulthood in families, in schools, on television, and throughout society are often negative. This is what the children absorb. Yet those young people who grow up relatively unencumbered by negative cultural models are able to handle people and situations with a sense of involvement, of enthusiasm, and of spontaneity.

I believe that a child lies dormant in every one of us, waiting to be recognized and accepted. It is natural for people to be happy, healthy, creatively alive, and childlike.

Yes, we are as young as we think, and the fountain of youth lies within each of us. We simply have to let ourselves shine each and every day as children do.

Some of you may be thinking that there's no way you can act like a child. You have a job with many responsibilities, you have bills to pay, and you have many problems and frustrations to deal with every day. But understand that children have problems and frustrations too. They have tests in school, difficulties with friends, and problems with parents, and yet they seem to bring a different attitude to life's situations. They handle things as they come up, without taking life so seriously. Young people can often show great wisdom. I'm not suggesting giving up adulthood. Rather, I suggest we integrate the child and the adult within us. That's the key to celebrating life.

One way of achieving this blend is to spend time around children. Watch them from afar. Play with them. Get involved. Throw yourself into their activities. Pretend you are a child again. Now if you don't have any children of your own, find a way to be with children at least once a month. You might do volunteer work with Big Sisters or Big Brothers, the Scouts, the local park, or the pediatric ward of a nearby hospital.

I know it will be valuable and worthwhile for you. Children have a way of revealing much to us about ourselves if we allow ourselves to be open to them. They are like mirrors, showing us many valuable lessons about living.

Following are a few of the lessons children have taught me.

Be All That You Can Be What a beautiful gift we can give to each other. Children know this well. Being all that you can be means being authentic, sensitive, vulnerable, and willing to express your feelings. When we're being who we are, we don't wear masks, we have no pretenses, we are ingenuous. Children exhibit these qualities when they meet a new friend. Even though they might start out with some shyness, when it feels right (and for children it almost always quickly becomes right), they relate as though they were long-time friends.

At my party three of the children were new to the neighborhood and didn't know anyone. Yet within the first few minutes they were all getting along as though they were best buddies.

Compare this approach with your own feelings and behavior when you meet someone new. How do you respond? How long is your initial period of shyness? Are you likely to feel reserved or suspicious? If you are, perhaps these feelings are related to how you feel about yourself. The ability to trust lies in your mind and is expressed through your attitude. In fact, what you believe to be true about yourself and about your world will be duplicated in all your life experiences. If you think the world is rotten, your world will reflect just that. If you think everyone is out to get you or use you, that's exactly the kind of people you will attract. Our thoughts have a great influence upon our circumstances.

In his marvelous book *Love*, Leo Buscaglia says this: "Love is like a mirror. When you love another you become his mirror and he becomes yours...and reflecting each other's love you see infinity." Yes, you are always in a relationship with yourself, especially in the presence of another. Acknowledge and be thankful to others for serving as your mirror.

The next time you meet a new person, be aware of your reactions. Notice if you are being cool, standoffish, keeping the person at arm's length with small talk. See if you are wondering what this person is after. Are you feeling a little uncomfortable, uncertain about where this new encounter is headed? If you are concerned about getting too involved, remember that your involvement need extend no further than this one meeting if you don't want it to. Take your cue from kids, who can have a great time together even if they know they may never see each other again. They are not averse to gaining something for fear of losing it. Set right out to find this new person's funnybone, or find some other way to put him or her at ease. When you show that you trust and respect someone, the barriers immediately begin to drop. If you let your childlike trust take over, and you feel positive about being able to handle anything that comes along, your very attitude of certainty will see you through.

A few years ago a friend and I went to see a play in Hollywood. After it was over, we decided to get a bite at a coffee shop down the street. It was late and there were few people in the restaurant. After awhile I noticed a ragged woman, who obviously didn't feel good about herself. The waitress told us that this woman came in every Saturday evening at the same time.

As I was visiting with my friend, I couldn't help but notice the woman's appearance. In her midfifties, she had dirty clothes and matted, greasy hair, and carried a backpack as her purse. I could sense her sadness and loneliness. I was keenly aware of my desire to reach out to her, but I didn't really know what to do.

My friend had to leave, but I decided to stay. I went over to the woman's table, touched her hand, and asked her to keep me company while I finished my meal. At that point she started to cry, and I thought to myself, Suze, you certainly misread your inner signals this time." As I sat down to try and mend the situation, this woman, Gloria, told me I was the first person to approach her with genuine warmth and caring in years!

Well, Gloria and I talked for an hour and she invited me to her apartment a couple blocks away. In her cramped and disheveled one-room apartment I listened through the night to her life story.

I found out that Gloria hadn't worked in more than a year and that, having no family, she rarely had visitors. As she spoke of her love for children, I remembered a telephone call I had received two weeks before. A friend who owns a day care center had called, asking me if I could recommend someone for an opening as a teacher's aide. I will never forget the sparkle in Gloria's eyes as I told her the details of this possible job.

Amazingly, it was now eight o'clock in the morning. I suggested she take a shower and then we could return to the coffee shop for breakfast. We also called the day care center owner. The position was still open, and I arranged for Gloria to have an interview later that day.

In the meantime, I helped Gloria curl her hair, showed her how to apply some makeup, and helped her to pick out a clean dress to wear for the interview. It was wonderful to see her transform before my eyes. As it turned out, Gloria got the job and began work the next week. After several weeks, I paid a surprise visit to Gloria at the center. I could hardly believe my eyes. She looked ten years younger and was aglow with enthusiasm. The children all loved her and so did the center's owner.

She invited me to her apartment for dinner that evening. I didn't recognize her home either. She had cleaned and painted every inch and even had a couple of plants on her dresser. I was so touched. Gloria was radiantly alive and happy, as she was meant to be. From this experience I truly learned the value of reaching out to another, even though you have no guarantee of the outcome. I believe that's what living is all about—person to person, heart to heart interchange. Participate in the adventure of life. With love in your heart and a willingness to risk and be vulnerable, all will be right. As the greatest teacher who ever lived said two thousand years ago, "Love thy neighbor as thyself."

This week go out and meet someone new. Introduce yourself to people, even if it feels funny at first. This will help shake off your inhibitions about talking to strangers. Trust new friends and yourself to make the best of the situation. Find out what it is you have in common. The more you do this, the more you'll discover, as I have, that what we have in common with each other far outweighs the differences, and further, that it's the differences that make friendships stimulating and exciting.

I had an illuminating experience last year as I was flying across country, coming home after a two-week lecture/TV tour. I was tired and needed to get some work done. I was hoping the seat next to me would be vacant, because I felt like being alone and not talking to anyone. No such luck. An elderly man sat down next to me and started talking a mile a minute. My inclination was to let him know I didn't feel like talking, yet my heart told me to simply listen and wait. With some resistance and some initial resentment, I quietly listened and learned a wonderful lesson that day. Brief encounters can be fantastic. Regardless of how long a friendship might last, whether a few minutes or a lifetime, each relationship is of value to the participants. I learned this man was a retired pilot and had flown everything from biplanes to supersonic stunt jets to ultralights. Because I love to fly and want to get my pilot's license one day, I delighted in five hours of stories and adventures I would not otherwise have had a chance to experience. And although I never saw him again, I'll always be grateful for our brief exchange and for recognizing the importance of sharing one to one with an open heart and acceptance.

The child in you knows how to deal with everyone and every situation with perfect aplomb. So allow your inner child to show you how to be a friend and how to make new friends.

It is also important to find ways to let your family and friends know you care. You don't have to wait for birthdays and anniversaries. Make every day Valentine's Day. If you have a difficult time expressing your feelings verbally, write a note, offer a hug, or send flowers. My Mom and I speak often by telephone. When we finish talking she always ends by telling me she loves me. That means so much to me. Remember too that just because a message might not be received or acknowledged the way you would wish, it's still worth sending. Live today as though it were your last day. Be that friend or loved one you would appreciate having.

Give Fantasy Its Wings And Fly Fantasy, or creative daydreaming, is a health experience for both children and adults. Remember how when you were a child your bedroom took on many worlds of its own? Sometimes it was a fortress, other times it was another planet. Remember when you dressed up or when you pretended you were a grocer, doctor, pilot, athlete, or ballet dancer? For both children and adults, creative dreaming provides a practical escape from the pressures of everyday living. It eliminates boredom and enhances creativity. And dreaming creates your reality; in fact, your present realities started with thoughts and dreams.

Children have the ability not to place limits on their thinking and dreaming. Anything and everything is possible for those who believe, and children understand this better than anyone. They possess limitless dreams and goals, and express their aspirations easily. I am saddened when I hear parents telling their children that it is silly to make up fantasies about pretend-friends or animals or trips out of the universe. Encourage your children to fantasize, and encourage them to share their dreams with you.

At my party four of the children gathered in the corner and had a great time visiting with E.T. on his own planet. It was so real and vivid to them.

To get back in touch with your fantasy life, you might try finding some children with whom to laugh and play, and encourage everyone to share his or her wildest dreams. You will discover how creative and spontaneous children can be, and it will rub off on you.

Give yourself permission to go out and enjoy some children's movies, a puppet show, an amusement park, or a circus. Take a couple of children with you. You'll have as much fun as the kids, perhaps more. Have you seen the Harlem Globetrotters in action? Each really knows how to let his or her inner child come out to play.

This week, go to your local playground and play. How long has it been since you've been on a swing? When was the last time you went barefoot in the sandbox? Have you ever thrown a frisbee or played tag with some kids? When was the last time you sat with some children to see who could make the funniest face?

What are some of your dreams and fantasies? Have you ever wanted to go sailing or windsurfing? Or how about river rafting or body surfing? Maybe you've wanted to paint, visit Nepal, learn aikido, bake bread, climb Mt. Whitney, or spend the night in the mountains. Whatever it is, make a list. It doesn't matter how crazy or silly these things may seem. You don't need to justify to anyone why you want to do these things. Just that you want to do something is reason enough to do it.

Now look over your list. Some things you wrote down will be difficult to do right away. But I'm sure that you listed at least one thing that you can do immediately. Do it today. Keep your list so that you can add to it as well as cross off things as you've accomplished them or changed your mind.

Acting out my fantasies has added enchantment and excitement to my life. Some of the things I've tried that are on my list include skydiving, hang gliding, motocross racing, painting, Tai Chi, photography, and camping alone in the mountains. Among the things still left on my list are to surf ski (ocean kayak) from Los Angeles to Catalina Island, swim along side a whale in the ocean, ride in a bi-plane, meet Michael Crawford and have him sing to me 'The Music of the Night' from Andrew Lloyd Weber's—The Phantom of the Opera.

Living In The Present

Our swaddled and weary senses restrain us in a mysterious land of suspension and removal which has the qualities of distance and separation. We let nothing really touch us and become slaves to automatic living, paying very little notice to what goes on around us. Thus, we deny ourselves the fullness of living in the now, which requires that we must be able to open fully our senses and to direct our awareness.
                                                —Herbert A. Otto, *Ways of Growth*

Living *in* the moment is different from living *for* the moment. Children allow themselves to get totally involved in and focused on whatever they are doing right now. Granted, their attention span is not long, but they are still able to focus on whatever is taking place in their lives at the moment. When they eat, they just eat; when they play, they just play; when they talk, they just talk. They throw themselves wholeheartedly into their activity. They are able to make whatever is happening to them at the moment okay.

I look back on my early childhood and recall that I had no sense of time. My family took frequent long trips in the car. Usually within ten minutes of leaving home I would ask, "Are we there yet?" followed by "When are we going to be there?" This was repeated every ten minutes or so. Two hours away didn't mean anything to me. My only sense of time was now.

I am not recommending we forget the future. I believe in planning ahead, preparing for the future, and fostering dreams. But that has its time and place. Most of the time, be here now. Be open to the touch, feelings, sights of what is around you and in you right now. Appreciate life with all of your senses.

I was reminded of the importance of being here now during my party when all the children were playing in the backyard. Although I came to the party feeling somewhat lugubrious, after only a few minutes I was so caught up in our activities and the fun we were all having that I didn't give a second thought to my disturbing telephone conversation. I was involved in having a wonderful time. If I had continued to think about the call, it would have taken away from my enjoyment of the party. We really can't live in the future or the past. Young children instinctively know this is a waste of time.

Have you ever noticed that children are willing to try anything at a moment's notice? Even though they might have experienced that same thing before, they will express wide-eyed excitement and wonderment. This is because children don't use a yardstick to measure activities or compare the present with the past. They know they've played the game before, or had someone read the same story just last night, yet it's still as fresh and as wonderful as it was the first time.

Think about your attitude when doing the dishes, vacuuming, or watering the plants. You probably find these activities boring. Have you ever seen a child help with the dishes or vacuum or water the plants? A child can't wait to participate, and acts as though it's just about the most exciting thing he or she has ever done. What a wonderful quality that is! To be excited about life—about every part of life—as though it's always fresh and new. Actually, it is. It's only old thoughts and distorted attitudes that cloud the eyes and get in the way of celebrating each moment.

Often when I'm conducting a workshop, I ask the participants to go outside for ten to fifteen minutes and saunter the grounds, alone, in silence. I have them practice being totally absorbed in what they can see, smell, taste, feel, and hear. To be with nature, letting its beauty into your awareness, is wonderful. What I have discovered in taking this kind of walk (and I do this at least once a week) is that I feel a subtle, gentle communion with nature. The flowers, trees, birds, even the insects seem to be in harmony with me. A delightful book called *Celebrate the Temporary*, by Clyde Reid has helped me to appreciate and live in the now. It's one of those books you'll want to share with your friends and family.

When was the last time you walked past a school playground when the children were playing? Make a point of doing this over the next few days. Notice how totally involved and absorbed the children are when they are playing. They seem oblivious to future problems and appear to have let go of annoyances of the past. They let their spontaneity run free. One moment they are totally involved with other children and participating in a certain game. Then, minutes later, they will change games and yet again be totally involved in another.

How spontaneous are you? If you are like many people, your schedule is tightly planned. It's appropriate to have goals, to make plans, to be disciplined with your time. But if you are too rigid, if your schedule is too strict, it will be hard for your inner child to come out and enjoy life. Plato's words, "Life must be lived as a play," are important to keep in mind.

I suggest that you set aside a specific time each day free from any scheduled activity. Then when the time rolls around, see what you feel like doing. How about daydreaming, writing a letter, going to the park, or taking a ride on your bike? Just ride and see where you end up. See what moves you at the moment. As you tune in more to your inner child, it will show you more and more how you can thoroughly enjoy each day and how being more spontaneous will add a new dimension to your life.

If your present is obscured by "if onlys," or "just wait until tomorrows," try the following exercise. Write down some of your self-limiting thoughts, beliefs, and habits. Take your time. Look deeply within. Include as many as you can think of. Then put your list in a brown paper bag. Close the top securely. Then, as you breathe deeply and slowly, put the bag in a fireplace and set it on fire. Watch all of your excess baggage dissolve before your eyes. Just let it go. And as it's dissolving, affirm something such as "I choose to embrace and celebrate life moment to moment."

Yesterday is a cancelled check: forget it. Tomorrow is a promissory note: don't count on it. Today is ready cash: use it!
—Edwin C. Bliss *Doing It Now*

Don't Be Afraid To Make Mistakes Or Fail Failure is only a word and has no power other than what you may give it. Children haven't yet learned the adult meaning of the word *failure* and thus have the desire to "go for it" most of the time. They take risks in life because they intuitively know that to risk is to learn and grow.

In going over some material I had on a well-known person I was surprised to read the following: He failed twice in business. He ran for the state legislature and for Congress, and he failed each time. He was also defeated two times in Senate races. Next he worked to become vice president of the United States, with no success. The love of his life died when she was very young. He suffered a nervous breakdown. But he didn't let his adversities and failures get the best of him. He eventually became president of the United States. His name is Abraham Lincoln. He once said, "Man is just about as happy as he makes up his mind to be." President Lincoln's courage and tenacity inspire all of us. He continued to risk and go after his dreams, without regard for appearances.

Have you ever watched a child learning to ride a bike? A child will try again and again, falling, getting up, and starting over, no matter how many times it takes, because he or she is not trying to prove anything to anyone else. A child isn't afraid of failing repeatedly in order to accomplish a goal. What is failure anyway? Just a delay in results.

Make a list of activities that you have avoided because they might look weird to others or because you were afraid you would fail. You might include learning to swim, play golf, dance, paint, ski, or sing. Or how about learning to play the piano or roller skate? Now how many of the activities on your list can you begin within the next couple of days? Start now!

At my party for children, we played a game that involved laying a large sheet of plastic on the ground. Then we turned on the hose and ran water over the plastic sheet. We ran and slid over it, twisting, spinning and getting entangled with each other. It was great fun and even though it was easy to slip and fall, as we all did, no one was concerned with how "foolish" he or she looked. We were all having a wonderful time enjoying the moment. Be more concerned with your own integrity and experience of living than what others might think.

Accept The World Just As It Is   Children don't resist life. They are incredibly accepting and have the unique ability to take things as they come, and make the most of them.

In adulthood we face many conditions that we wish were different—all the way from world hunger, environmental pollution, and rising prices to our fitness routine or diet. Many times, no matter what we do, things don't seem to change fast enough. The key is to get involved, while trying to keep a clear perspective of the situation. Do this without getting angry or upset at the challenging situation. As the beautiful Serenity Prayer says,

> Lord, give me the strength to change those things that can be changed, to accept those things that cannot be changed, and the wisdom to know the difference.

Children seem to have a natural understanding of this.

Take the weather. It's clearly a natural phenomenon that we cannot control. Let's say it's early morning and you've just woken up. You discover that it snowed heavily all night. The roads are a mess and your driveway is full of snow. You begin bemoaning your fate, dreading your drive to work. Even if you choose to stay home, you've already convinced yourself that the day is wasted. The children on the other hand, haven't been this excited in days. Either they'll get to walk through the snow to school or, if they stay home, they'll be able to play all day in this white winter wonderland. What heaven!

Last week a friend of mine had plans to play tennis. Instead, Mother Nature decided to bless us with some much-needed rain. His tennis plans were ruined. Yet instead of finding a way to celebrate the wetness, he chose to sulk around his house all day, being angry at the weather. What a waste of life time!

You see, it's all just a matter of your attitude. Make whatever is going on in your life at the moment okay. Accept what is and what can't be changed, and make the best of it.

Be in touch with your emotions, express yourself, complete your emotions, and then let them go. Babies do this so marvelously. Think back to the last time you saw a baby be really upset. (For some of you, that might be within the past hour.) A baby will cry his or her heart out, will purely express his or her upset. When a baby's crying, I doubt that the baby's wondering if he or she should be crying and probably doesn't feel guilty or embarrassed for crying. The baby purely cries, then lets it go. Similarly, when a baby's angry, he or she will let you know and will also quickly let it go without holding onto it or holding resentment. Babies express themselves fully, then move on. What delightful teachers and what a perfect demonstration of the positive use of energy they are!

It occurs to me as I'm sitting here writing this that all these magical qualities I'm discussing in this chapter that are expressed by children and babies are also shared by animals. Perhaps that's why I've always been a great lover of animals, especially dogs, cats, horses, and birds.

It has been my experience that when I'm not accepting the circumstances in my life, I tend to try to be more controlling of people and situations instead of letting go and being in the flow of life. Yet as I choose to release my desire to be in control, I notice that the struggle dissipates and I feel more peaceful and joyous about myself and life. The more I pay attention to how children and animals experience and embrace life, and the more I release my fears about being rejected and feeling uncertain, the better life becomes for me and for those people around me, because I become softer and kinder.

Robert Mack, M.D., whom I introduced in Chapter 2, said this about being more in the flow of life.

> I have come to realize that there is a controlling self within me that is rigid, demanding, and judgmental. Life flows far better for me and for those around me when I am able to replace that person with a more caring, gentle me. When I can forgive and forget, when I can say and feel that whatever has happened is acceptable, when I can

take people in my arms and embrace them and be embraced and discover that we are each special, unique, and wondrous, then life becomes a great river that will flow no matter what I do. I can flow with it and live in peace or I can slip back into old patterns and live in despair, fighting against the current. The river does not care. It only makes a difference to me and to those around me. The choice is mine. The struggle to be a different person, to respond differently to life and to the people I know, is not a change I made once and now worry about no more. It is an ongoing struggle to be more soft and flexible, to give myself permission to enjoy who I am and what I do, to allow myself to laugh, tease, and relax in undemanding ways that really feel good. When I am successful in allowing those things to happen, my life is better for me and far better for the people around me.

I don't know about you, but when I read that, I get goose bumps. To live as this paragraph suggests, I believe, would change the world, would create a world of peace, harmony, and everlasting joy.

Laugh And Be A Little Silly When was the last time you really laughed? If you can't remember, you had better read this carefully, because your life might depend on it. Laughter is the lubricant of life. It's the elixir that enables you to experience the fullness and joy of life. Science is now discovering that there are salutary benefits from laughing.

Along with laughter comes smiling. Smile more. And if you need some reasons why, I'll give you a few: (1) it's great for firming your facial muscles; (2) it makes you feel better; (3) it makes people wonder what you've been up to; and (4) it's the shortest distance between two people.

Concomitant with laughter is not taking yourself or life too seriously. In *A Separate Reality*, Carlos Casteneda said something significant, namely, that a person of knowledge understands that what he or she does doesn't really matter, but he or she acts as though it does. So that when a wise person finishes what he or she has set out to do, whether it worked or it didn't is insignificant to that individual. The wise person is at peace knowing that everything is just perfect the way it is.

Being able to laugh at yourself and the incongruities of every-day situations is the best way to quell stress and to enjoy life. Three weeks ago this idea came alive for me. I took my car to the local automatic car wash. After paying, I came back outside and noticed that my car was parked separately from all the others. A few other car owners and most of the car wash employees were standing around my car, some looking shocked, some gesturing wildly, and some laughing. At first I thought they were admiring my good-looking automibile. As I got closer I saw what all the excitement was about. I had forgotten to close the sun roof and there was a lake inside my car! It was then that I noticed a huge sign on the wall that read, "Close all windows and sun roofs." I hesitantly opened the car door. And then it struck me how funny this all was, and I began laughing so hard my stomach hurt. Well, as I sit here relating my story, my car is almost dry. It would have done no good to get upset, and besides I am now driving a car with the cleanest interior for miles around. I had often wondered what it would be like to leave the sun roof open in a car wash. And now I know.

This is a good spot to remind you to watch your thoughts and wishes. You eventually get what you request.

Laugh! Laugh! Laugh! And do it often each day.

Children are special in this way. They intuitively realize that happiness is a choice—an attitude they create. That's why children often act silly and crazy, making and telling jokes. They also know how to cultivate a sense of humor, which, in my estimation, is one of the most important components of wellness.

In Viktor E. Frankl's book *Man's Search for Meaning,* he tells the story of his experiences in the Nazi concentration camps. In this poignant account he discusses the importance of humor to well-being and to staying alive. This is what he says. "Humor was another of the soul's weapons in the fight for self-preservation. It is well known that humor, more than anything else in the human make-up, can afford an aloofness and ability to rise above any situation, even if only for a few seconds."

So let your inner child come out and play. When you do, you find it natural and easy to look for the good in every person and in every situation, no matter what the appearances. Keep laughing your way through life. As Norman Cousins says in his marvelous book *The Anatomy of An Illness*, "Laughter is the best medicine." You don't always have to be orderly and serious.

Learn to laugh, especially at yourself! Give yourself permission to have fun and be a little giddy. In other words, lighten up. When you do this the world will seem brighter and more beautiful. Children have so much to teach us in this area.

Too often we get all bothered by what we perceive as important issues, and we forget that what's truly essential is invisible to the eye. This idea came alive for me when I read *The Little Prince* by St. Exúpery, the story of a prince who lives on an asteroid and doesn't know anything about love. One day he encounters a rose that's beautiful but vain. She causes him much suffering. So he sets off to learn about love and meets a wise little fox, who teaches him that people are so involved in matters of consequence that they forget what is essential. For what is essential is seen only with the heart; it is invisible to the eye.

Each day be a little crazy. Write a silly note and hide it in one of the shoes or pockets of a family member so he or she will find it later. Throw snowballs, fly a kite, hug a tree, skip pebbles over the water, kiss a flower and rub it against your face, bring home a birthday cake even though it's nobody's birthday, talk to a butterfly, or record a made-up song and send it to a friend. Let go of wondering what other people will think of you. It doesn't matter. What matters is that you enjoy being with you and that you have lots of fun in your own company. When you do, other people will too.

Every once in awhile, a few friends and I go on an adventure I call a Surprise Run. The group of us start out from some point and go for a run. Every time we get to the next corner, one runner gets to pick where to go next—straight, turn right, turn left, or maybe about face. We never know where the run will take us; it's all a surprise. Then the person who chose the direction for that block must also choose one surprise adventure on that block, which can be just about anything. Some of the things I've suggested are petting animals, picking up scattered garbage, watching birds, and imitating birds. Crazy, you say. Perhaps.

Other special times for me occur four times a year, during the change of seasons. These four high-energy days I celebrate by doing things such as lighting candles and buying flowers, both reflecting the season's colors. I dance and sing for the sun and moon. I make special gifts and offer these to Mother Nature. (I also celebrate the full and new moons.) Sure, I've had more than a few people tell me that I'm definitely crazy. I take their remark as a compliment and celebrate it. You see, it gives me great leeway for oddball behavior.

Love Unconditionally To me, the ability to love unconditionally is the most precious quality within us. All life is positively affected by love. Love is an unlimited source of energy and serves as the basic foundation of all life, of all joy. Along with love come the gifts of kindness, tenderness, forgiveness, and service. Lao Tzu, the great Chinese philosopher, once said, "Kindness in words creates confidence, kindness in thinking creates profoundness, and kindness in giving creates love."

A child's love is the perfect example of these God-given qualities. Have you noticed that children quickly forget their anger and forgive others when they've been hurt? Children accept you totally for your good points and for your not-so-good points too. They don't care about differences in people—about different races, religions, or backgrounds. They just love. In exchange, they are lovable, for that's exactly what they attract to themselves. The more we love, the more we are loved and the lovelier we are. We attract to ourselves the equivalent of that which we believe and express. Children are prepared to accept people as people, and even if offended or hurt, children will come back to forgive and love over and over again.

Part of loving another unconditionally is serving that person with your true attention and real feelings, and listening to his or her feelings. What a beautiful gift this is—to listen to the other person's hurt, anger, and upset without getting defensive. Be receptive, not reactive. That's the key.

If you tend to hold on to past resentments or grudges toward other people, examine your feelings. This is especially important with regard to negative feelings toward parents. Unresolved conflicts with or old bitterness toward your parents will interfere with your other relationships, especially your most intimate relationships. An excel-

lent book on this topic is *Making Peace With Your Parents,* by Harold
Bloomfield, M.D.

Children have helped me see more clearly that relationships work
best when we offer forgiveness to everyone. It is often difficult for
us to see the projection process within ourselves, and it's even more
difficult to stop our projections. But when we practice forgiveness,
all our relationships begin to change.

Because of a child's loving and forgiving nature, he or she tends
to be naturally grateful for life's treasures. A few weeks ago I finished a tour of schools of all levels, where I presented lectures and
workshops entitled "Health Power" and "Wellness Lifestyling." In
one particular school I worked with children aged four to eight. I
asked them what made them feel grateful. Here are some of the
responses I received. "I'm grateful to be breathing, because my breath
gives me life." (She was five.) "I'm grateful for my birthdays, because
that's a day I give my parents presents for bringing me into the
world." (He was eight.) "I'm grateful for my cat. When she purrs
I know she's happy, and that makes me happy." (She was six.) "I'm
grateful for my new bike, because I love to feel the wind on my face
and hair when I ride. I also like to share my bike with my best friend,
because she doesn't have a bike yet." (She was seven.)

DECIDE TO FORGIVE

Decide to forgive
For resentment is negative
Resentment is poisonous
Resentment diminishes
and devours the self.
Be the first to forgive,
To smile and to take the first step,
And you will see happiness bloom
On the face of your human
brother or sister.
Be always the first
Do not wait for others to forgive

For by forgiving
You become the master of fate
The fashioner of life
The doer of miracles.
To forgive is the highest,
most beautiful form of love.
In return you will receive
untold peace and happiness.

—Robert Muller

The former assistant secretary-general of the United Nations wrote this poem for International Forgiveness Week, held annually.

The qualities of unconditional love and forgiveness are taught beautifully in *A Course in Miracles*. When we begin reacting to others with the understanding that they are Spirit—one with ourselves and all others—we realize that nothing their physical body says or does can truly hurt us.

The quality of unconditional love was made clearer to me the day of my neighborhood party. Just before it was over, I saw two small girls hugging and kissing each other. Just five minutes earlier they had been angry at each other because one of the girls had taken the last piece of carrot cake. Without any interference by me or the other children, I watched the two girls handle their problem. One girl decided to share the piece of cake, and the other girl thanked her with a big hug and kiss. I was very touched by the girls' generosity. Later I called my friend with whom I had the disagreement, to say that I was sorry for the misunderstanding and also to say "I love you." It was easy and natural, and I felt grateful to those two little girls for showing me how to express my love more freely and unconditionally.

I believe with all my heart that in a world where so much conflict exists between people of different races, religions, and backgrounds, the greatest bridge to understanding and peace is laughter and love. It's through compassion, forgiveness, laughter, and love that we can create a world where everyone wins, where everyone lives in peace and harmony. Never underestimate the power of love; it is the solution to any problem.

Children know this better than most of us. Watch them. Learn from them.

Let's all begin today to live more joyfully, to play at the game of life. Let the child within you blossom. Permit yourself to experience life to its fullest—to celebrate you and life.

Learn from children that the elixir for perpetual youth lies within every one of us. Each day is a brand new rainbow full of love, joy, wonder, and celebration.

> Someday, after we have mastered the winds, the waves, the tides and gravity, we shall harness for God the energies of love. Then for the second time in the history of the world, man will have discovered fire.
> —Teilhard de Chardin

Self-Discovery Questions

1. *In what areas of my life am I too serious?*

2. *Would I describe myself as a happy, positive person? Am I the type of person I would like to have for a friend?*

3. *How do I feel being around children?*

4. *What qualities do I see in children that I'd like to integrate more fully into my life?*

5. *In what areas of my life am I too rigid and orderly—too "adult"?*

6. *Do I give myself permission to act silly and crazy?*

7. *How often do I truly embrace the moment? Do I spend my present moments feeling guilty about the past or worrying about the future?*

Action Choices

1. *If I were to regularly let the child in me out to explore, play, be spontaneous, and be creative, my life would change in the following ways:*

2. *In order to get more in touch with my inner child, I am going to spend some time observing children at play as well as participating with them. I can do this in the following ways:*

3. *Following are fun things to do for those I care about (for example, write a special note, send flowers, or record a song):*

4. *Here are some things I tried in the past six months that I had never tried before:*

5. *Here are some new ventures I choose to undertake in the coming six months:*

6. *Here are some changes I can make to become a little less serious, to lighten up:*

7. *The following are people I have wanted to meet or get to know better. I'll choose one of them to get together with next week.*

8. *Following is a description of myself as a happy, positive, magnificent person:*

9. *Each day I'll set some time aside to envision my ideal life. I will now spend the next few moments imagining one of my goals as already achieved. Here is what I visualized that to be:*

Let us then pursue what makes for peace and for mutual upbuilding.
—Romans 14:19

Change yourself and you have done your part in changing the world. Every individual must change his own life if he wants to live in a peaceful world. The world cannot become peaceful unless and until you yourself begin to work toward peace.
—Paramahansa Yogananda

The most significant contribution you and I can make toward world peace is to be peaceful ourselves, to give peacefulness to those whose lives we touch daily, and to forgive ourselves for our errors, to the point at which we love ourselves no matter what we have ever done.
—John R. Price, The Quartus Report #10, 1986

One day the people of the world will want peace so much that the governments are going to have to get out of their way and give it to them.
—President Dwight D. Eisenhower

Peace between countries must rest on the solid foundation of love between individuals.
—Mahatma Gandhi

CHAPTER 7

CHOOSE

A PEACEFUL, POSITIVE ATTITUDE

Everything can be taken from a man but one thing: the last of the human freedoms—to choose one's attitude in any given set of circumstances, to choose one's own way.

Viktor E. Frankl,
Man's Search for Meaning

Attitude—this has to do with your mind, how you look at life, and what you express. William James, the noted philosopher, put it concisely when he said, "The greatest discovery of our generation is that a human being can alter his life by altering his attitude."

Yes, our attitude about life has everything to do with whether we are happy or sad, successful or unsuccessful, filled with joy or with feelings of disease. Certainly situations arise in our lives that seem difficult, but the healthiest attitude is to see problems only as opportunities to grow and evolve. In the evolution of consciousness, our greatest problem is always our richest opportunity. That is to say, nothing happens in life that does not afford some value.

You have more strength to overcome difficulties than you have troubles to overcome.

Last week I was in Palm Springs lecturing, and one of the participants told me about a woman whom she had recently interviewed for a magazine. Her story is a perfect, inspiring example of finding opportunity in problems.

Marilyn Hamilton was a teacher and beauty queen. When she was 29 years old, she had an accident while hang gliding: she fell down a rocky cliff that left her in a wheelchair, paralyzed below the waist. Instead of seeing herself as a victim, she chose to see her accident as an opportunity. And because she felt too restricted in her wheelchair, she designed a better one. She now has a business called Motion Designs, which is a multimillion-dollar success story that revolutionized the wheelchair industry and went on to become California's Small Business of the Year for 1984.

If we could see the whole picture, if we could grasp the entire story, we would realize that no problem ever comes to us that does not have a purpose in our life. All so-called problems contribute to our inner growth.

A few years ago I trained to be an Emergency Medical Technician. For about a year I occasionally volunteered in emergency rooms of local hospitals. One day's experiences will forever be vivid in my mind as among my saddest and most poignant. It was Christmas Day and, for awhile, the emergency room was quiet. One patient with a sprained ankle and another with a severe stomachache were the only cases. Then, all at once, three more patients came: three attempted suicides. Two made it through; the third didn't. I had an opportunity to visit with the two survivors, a woman and a man. The thoughts and beliefs of both were much the same. The woman had experienced several painful relationships, which led her to withdraw to protect herself. She was unable to recognize that she had other choices. She was unwilling to risk more pain. The man had lost his job and felt worthless as a human being. He felt that there must be something better somewhere, but not here on Earth. They both dreaded pain and did whatever they could to avoid it. They didn't understand that to live without pain is to be only half-alive.

Choose to live in the full spectrum of wholeness. Suppose you see a rainbow. You notice one or two colors you don't like. But would it be a rainbow without all the colors blending with one another? Similarly, all that's taking place in your life is what you've asked for or needed, even if you don't realize it. And it's your thoughts about and attitude toward what is happening that make the difference. Let go of judgment. Understand that what takes place in the present does not have to be a duplication of your past.

So with a new willing, positive attitude, you will come to understand that it is not the times, complications of society, or other people that cause our problems; it is only our inability to cope with the times, complications, and people. In other words, *it's not what's happening—it's how you take it*. Or as Shakespeare put it, "There is nothing either good or bad, but thinking makes it so." Make whatever is going on with you at the moment okay. We must celebrate our pain; celebrate our insecurities; celebrate every experience we have. This proves we are alive. And it's through our willingness to let go, to risk, to experience living that we learn, grow, and become stronger. As Emerson says, "Our strengths grow from our weakness."

Realize that everything in the universe is just as it should be. The evidence: it is. Live in this moment. Be fascinated by and embrace the present. Every single moment has something special to offer. Something beautiful. But it's up to us to discover it.

Take hold of life. Most of the things that distress you, you can avoid; many of the things that dominate you, you can overthrow. You can do as you like with them.

—Plato

We develop according to that upon which our mind dwells, and we attract to ourselves the equivalent of that which we express— what we think, visualize, and affirm. Negative thinking and a negative attitude inhibit the flow of positive energy through you and cause disharmonies of the body, mind, and spirit. Criticism, anger, envy, suspicion, fear, hate, doubt, laziness, worry, guilt, feelings of worthlessness, and so on are all forms of negation. Watch your thoughts! Stop them from pointless wandering; make them obey you. Train your mind to think constructively and positively at all times, regardless of appearances. This also means to pay attention to what comes out of your mouth; your words are as important as what you think and feel.

To recapitulate, the thoughts we hold determine our experience. In other words, what we experience is our attitude or state of mind projected outward. If our state of mind is one of wellness, joy, and love, that is what we will project and therefore experience. If we are filled with thoughts of fear, worry, doubt, or concern about illness, we will project this state outward, and it will become our reality.

Thought is the substance from which all things are created. Your tomorrows are designed by your thoughts today. Take charge today, this moment. You live in exquisite freedom of will to accept and embrace whatever thoughts you choose. You are the creator, the architect of your life. And with this awesome power, you create everything for yourself. In the silence of our being, we possess the ability to think, the ability to feel, and the ability to create and become whatever we want to become. This very moment we are all precisely what we have chosen to be.

Start with loving and embracing yourself, for this is the way to peace and happiness. Loving yourself fully and unconditionally will give you the love to embrace the whole of humanity.

Next, if you are harboring the slightest resentment, bitterness, or unkind thought toward anyone, work at letting it go immediately. Your negative thoughts are only hurting you. In his marvelous book *Good-Bye to Guilt*, Gerald Jampolsky, M.D., says, "We cannot demonstrate total love until we have healed all of our relationships." Hate injures the hater more than the hated.

Strive to live all the healthy things you believe in. *When what you think, feel, say, and do is in harmony, you will know peace.*

Once when Gandhi's train was pulling out of a station, someone ran up to his window and asked to be given some helpful message. To that, Gandhi answered, "My life is my message."

Next, take your positive attitude and give it away. Brighten another's day. Spread joy. Offer kindness to others. You know, it's really quite simple. All people want in life is some love, some attention, and some respect. With the right attitude, we can find ways to give these each day. And the beauty is that it costs nothing and that your life is enriched also.

Yes, a joyful, thankful attitude will carry you a long way toward the goal of bringing into your life the good that you desire and deserve. Let your attitude be one of joining, not separating, yourself from other people and from life. When you carry around a feeling of separateness you see yourself as being at the center of the universe, and tend to judge everything as it relates to you. As a human being you are a valuable cell in the body of humanity, not separate from your fellow humans. It's only from this higher viewpoint and attitude that you can know what it is to love your neighbor as yourself. It is from this perspective that you can come to realize that everything you express affects the universe.

This attitude of treating yourself and others with respect and dignity will not only enrich your life but can also enhance the success of a business. In the book *In Search of Excellence,* authors Thomas J. Peters and Robert H. Waterman, Jr., set out to discover what factors made companies great. They found that one of the factors was a passionate attention to people. "There was hardly a more pervasive theme in excellent companies than respect for the individual," they wrote. Further, they said that the companies that succeeded were the ones that treated people with respect and dignity, and treated their employees as partners, rather than tools.

When you are happy, the world is more happy. When you are depressed, the world reacts to that depression. When you are well and vibrantly alive, the world is made more healthy. Likewise, when you feel sick, the world is more challenged. This wholeness viewpoint is summarized beautifully in these two poems:

To see the world in a grain of sand
And heaven in a wildflower
Hold infinity in the palm of your hand
And eternity in an hour.

—William Blake

We are one, after all, you and I, together
we suffer, together exist.
And forever will recreate each other.

                                        —Teilhard de Chardin

Clearly, no man, no woman is an island. We are one family. And you are important to the health and well-being of the world. How you choose to live your life makes a difference. No matter who you are, what color your skin, where you live, what you do for a living, what form of worship you practice, you are a unique and magnificent human being and the world is better because of you. You can elect to enrich the quality of all life even more by how you choose to live your life. I love what Emerson once said about living successfully: "To leave the world a bit better, whether by a healthy child, a garden patch or a redeemed condition, to know that even one life breathed easier because you lived, this is to have succeeded." And George Bernard Shaw, whose life spanned almost one hundred years, said so lovingly as he reflected on his life,

> I am convinced that my life belongs to the whole community; and as long as I live, it is my privilege to do for it whatever I can, for the harder I work the more I live. I rejoice in life for its own sake. Life is no brief candle for me. It is a sort of splendid torch which I got hold of for a moment, and I want to make it burn as brightly as possible before turning it over to future generations.

It starts with you—your attitude, your feelings, your thoughts, and your words. Take a good look at your life, and if you want to change it, change your attitude, feelings, thoughts, and words. Because you alone are responsible for them, only you can change them.

It is a matter of choice. It is always an inside job. Blaming others for your circumstances in life is always off course.

> People are always blaming their circumstances for what they are. I don't believe in circumstances. The people who get on in this world are the people who get up and look for the circumstances they want and if they can't find them, make them.
>
>   —George Bernard Shaw

In *As A Man Thinketh*, James Allen says the same thing, but from a different perspective.

> Of all the beautiful truths pertaining to the soul which have been restored and brought to life in this age, none is more gladdening or fruitful of divine promise and confidence than this—that man is the master of thought, the moulder of character, and the maker and shaper of condition, environment and destiny.

Yes, wellness is only a thought away. Paradise is only a thought away. This new attitude begins with our beliefs and words about ourselves and life. I believe that all the outside factors, including diet, exercise, work, relationships, and so on, are of little value until we learn to live in peace and harmony with ourselves and our environment. As Emerson says, "What lies behind us and what lies before us are tiny matters compared to what lies within us."

For me, finding peace goes hand in hand with some other qualities that are part of wellness. These include laughter, meditation, deep breathing, not taking life so seriously, living in the present, simplifying, and expressing serenity.

One of the most difficult journeys we ever have to take is the eighteen inch journey from the head to the heart. As we live more from our hearts (from love) and less from our heads (analyzing, criticizing, and judging), we will "lighten up." It will be easier to look for the good in every person and situation. We'll be able to bring harmony into any unpeaceful situation. Insofar as we have peace and love in our hearts, we reflect it into our surroundings and into our world.

"Most of the shadows in life are caused by standing in our own sunshine," says Emerson. So lighten up, let your heart light shine. When you do that, you'll understand what joy there is in embracing each day, in living right here in the present.

We can't really live in the past or the future, but we can unfortunately squander our present moments regretting the past and worrying about the future. Worry is such a waste of time. This negative emotion inhibits us from living in the present moment. Worry is different from concern. Concern motivates you to do everything possible to change a situation. Worry is a useless mulling over of things you cannot change. We agonize over the past, which we should let go of, or we're apprehensive about the future, which hasn't-arrived yet. All we ever have is this present moment, and if you don't live it, you never really get around to living at all. As *A Course in Miracles* says, "Look lovingly upon the present, for it holds the only things that are forever true."

It is my experience that when one goes beyond thinking that one must or should do this or that, and gets down to the business—or joy—of being, living in the moment, one experiences a magnificent happiness and a greater freedom than one has ever known before—a surrender into life and how it is meant to be lived. That is our purpose: to be! We're a human being, not a human doing.

What if in the present moment you feel upset or depressed? Immediately take your mind off of your thoughts and visions of what you don't want, and put it on thoughts and visions of what you *do* desire. Also, keep your surroundings harmonious, with beautiful music and lovely flowers. Read spiritual and uplifting books and magazines that inspire and motivate you. Make a list of the things for which to be grateful. If there is something you've always wanted to do, do it now. Find ways you can be of service to others. Following these suggestions will make your present moments come alive and shine brightly.

Every moment is a special gift to us from God, and what we do with each moment is our gift to God.

> What is the use of planning to be able to eat next week unless I can really enjoy the meals when they come? If I am so busy planning how to eat next week that I cannot fully enjoy what I am eating now, I will be in the same predicament when next week's meals become "now".
>
> If my happiness at this moment consists largely in reviewing happy memories and expectations, I am but dimly aware of this present. I shall still be dimly aware of the present when the good things that I have been expecting come to pass. For I shall have formed a habit of looking behind and ahead, making it difficult for me to attend to

PEACEFUL, POSITIVE ATTITUDE

the here and now. If, then, my awareness of the past and future makes me less aware of the present, I must begin to wonder whether I am actually living in the real world.

Alan W. Watts, *The Wisdom of Insecurity*

This very moment is sacred. It is the culmination of past good and a preview of infinite and even greater good. It is the present moment, the new day, an opportunity to love. And it brings with it power and glory. Unfortunately, it often takes a major calamity, a life-threatening disease or a near-death experience, for many people to truly experience living in the moment, to appreciate the beauty, wonder, and magnificence of life. A peak experience can force us into being right in the moment. And when it's over, quite often our life changes, takes on new meaning and purpose. Life emerges anew; priorities change and what was once mundane—say a breeze or a cloud—suddenly becomes exciting. Living becomes a passionate adventure. The subtle beauty of life reaches out and enfolds us and we, in turn, embody the sparkle of life. I have seen this vividly with a few friends who found out they had only a short time left to live. Hearing this, they chose to live life to the fullest—which is exactly what living is all about.

Don't waste any time. Don't wait for a catastrophe. If you knew you were about to die, you'd start right this moment to enjoy life. You would not waste time on fear, lethargy, or trying to earn awards or recognition. You'd find ways to be happy, without reason, just for the sheer pleasure of it. You'd become fully responsible for your life, enabling you to be fully human. And you'd come to understand the truth of the popular song:

Row, row, row your boat, gently down the stream,
Merrily, merrily, merrily, merrily,
Life is but a dream.

Live today, not as though it were the first day of the rest of your life, but rather as though it were the last day.

Understand that you don't have to have an experience of being right on the edge of life to decide to live more fully. You can make that choice right now. Right this moment. *You can choose to see things differently, to live life from love, peace, and joy instead of fear.*

Several months ago I had a glorious experience that reminded me to "be here now" and to celebrate living each day. It also clearly showed me the tremendous power of thought.

It was a splendid morning and, as I like to do each week, I went to the beach for an invigorating swim. It was very early, just before sunrise. After some stretching exercises and a short run, I was ready for my swim. Because it was the end of summer, the water was still comfortably warm. But this morning there was something in the air that I couldn't quite put my finger on. I felt it deep inside me—a joyful anticipation, a faint knowing that today would be different, that this day would be one I would celebrate the rest of my life. I went out into the ocean, rode a few waves, and then swam past the swells.

I was aware of the peacefulness of the water. Glassy, sparkling, and clear, it rejuvenated my body and soul with each stroke. A few minutes later some old friends joined me, a group of pelicans who seem to enjoy escorting me. They were gliding flawlessly a few feet above my head when suddenly they flew away. Surprised, I waved good-bye as I turned over to begin the backstroke. It was then that I saw something that made my heart plummet.

About two weeks before this swim I had watched an incredible PBS special on sharks. The images and feeling from that program were still vivid in my mind. Then a few days after that, I had watched a moving Jacques Cousteau special about dolphins. For as long as I can remember, I have had a deep love for dolphins and whales.

Following the dolphin show, during my evening meditation, I visualized myself swimming and playing with a school of dolphins. I accepted and affirmed that that was my desire and reality. I then thanked God for this wonderful experience.

It was now only a few days later, and here I was starting the backstroke part of my swim when, off in the distance, I spotted a large, dark, frightening fin heading straight for me. My instant thought was—shark! I quickly looked toward the beach. No one was there. I had always taken for granted that I would stay calm in a life-threatening situation. But not this time! I can laugh now, but you should have seen me that morning. As the fin continued in my direction, I simply froze and tread water. I was so terrified, I couldn't even cry or swim away. And then it happened, a sight that will forever warm my heart and soul. The fin danced out of the water. It was a dolphin followed by a school of about two dozen more!

For the next half hour the dolphins stayed with me, swimming, jumping out of the water, and jumping over me. I swam underwater with them, listening to their beautiful sounds, touching their skin, feeling an exchange of love. For what seemed like hours, nothing else existed except my world of dolphins. I was oblivious to any thought of the past or future. Being right in the moment, I rejoiced in the joy of discovery.

Then, as quickly as they had arrived, they swam off, and I was left alone and immensely grateful. I swam back to the shore, where there was now a group of people who had gathered and watched my dance with the dolphins. I answered many questions and tried to share what the experience had been like for me. I found it was very hard to put my feelings into words. Experiences that speak directly to your heart are often difficult to express clearly.

The others left and I just sat there, enveloped in wonder at this truly remarkable experience. All I could do was cry—what had happened touched me so deeply, so lovingly.

Because of that experience I can never doubt the power of thought to create any reality we choose. The experience also was a beautiful lesson in living in the present and appreciating each moment.

There are times when we are living in the present, however, but are unable to experience and enjoy it fully because so much is going on. Do you try to read while eating, talk on the phone while listening to the radio, or exercise while watching TV? I call that PMO—present moment overload. Concentrate on doing one thing at a time. If you are eating a meal, do just that. How often as we profess to be listening to someone else are we thinking of many other

things? One of the greatest acts of love and kindness we can show
someone is simply to pay attention, to really be there with the other
person. We were born with two ears and one mouth; maybe God
was trying to tell us something. Simplify your thoughts when you
are with another. Again, it's that eighteen-inch journey from the
head to the heart.

Simplify. What a wonderful word and a powerful process this
is. I have discovered great joy in simplifying all areas of my life. This
includes my thoughts, what I say, how I choose to spend my
time—and my closets, cupboards, and garage! It is so freeing and
feels so good to simplify. For example, look at the foods you eat in
one meal. It's hard to appreciate any one of them fully when there's
so many mixed together. Similarly, you can have a fantastic collec-
tion of art objects in your home, but if there's too many—if it's
cluttered—then it is difficult to appreciate each piece fully.

Henry David Thoreau says:

> An honest man has hardly need to count more than his ten fingers,
> or in extreme cases he may add his ten toes, and lump the rest. Sim-
> plicity, Simplicity, Simplicity. I say, let your affairs be as two or three,
> and not a hundred or a thousand; instead of a million, count half-a-
> dozen, and keep your affairs on your thumbnail.

Simplifying your life can be a wonderful experience. Simplicity
is to your soul what a detoxification program is to your body. They
both purify, yet simplicity is often difficult for a confused mind to
appreciate. What can you do to simplify your life right now, today?
You could start with cleaning out and simplifying one of your
closets, some cupboards, or one corner of your garage. Perhaps you
can do two or three cupboards a day until you have finished with
your entire house. What you'll discover, as a result, is that you will
find yourself more easily and naturally beginning to simplify other
areas of your life—how you spend your time, what you think, and
what you say. And this will not only be a freeing and refreshing
experience, but it will support you in feeling more serene. It was
Gandhi who said, "Live Simply so that others may Simply Live."

I have also noticed that concomitant with the process of simplification is the desire for slowing down and letting go of the need to always be in a hurry. There's an American sickness I've seen growing over the past ten years that I call a hurry-sickness. We see it everywhere. Instant breakfasts, fast foods, in-and-out cleaners, one-minute managers, twelve-minute fitness programs. I wouldn't be surprised to soon see a new book about "one-minute sex." Slow down, breathe deeply, and celebrate each day, each moment without rushing.

Serenity is the ability to enjoy life, to be happy and fulfilled, and to be at peace with yourself and your world. It's the result of unifying with your Higher Self, with the light and love within. It's not about arriving, for we have already arrived. And it's not about acquiring things. It has to do with just being content. Contentment is not the acquiring of things you desire, but rather the realization of what you already have and are. So being serene has to do with simply being who you are—the gift, the miracle.

One of the masters of the art of serenity was Thomas Edison. When his factory burned down, he did not bemoan his fate. As newspaper reporters came to interview him immediately following the disaster, they found him calmly at work on plans for a new building. It is also noted that he said of his deafness that it was an asset, because from it he learned to listen to what was within.

Helen Keller, a remarkable, inspiring woman who lived her life in deafness and blindness, also knew the joy of serenity. She said, "I learned that it is possible for us to create light and sound and order within us no matter what calamity may befall us in the outer world."

Mother Theresa is another human being who embodies serenity and peacefulness. So simply and lovingly she says, "Listen to the silence of your heart."

According to Webster's dictionary, serenity is the quality or state of being serene—calm, tranquil, peaceful, quiet, noiseless. To master the art of serenity, perhaps we need to master another art, that of solitude—being alone and finding peace in our own company. How do you feel about spending time alone? Aloneness is different from loneliness. This idea is expressed beautifully by Paul Tillich in his book *Courage To Be*. He says, "Our language has wisely sensed the two sides of being alone. It has created the word *loneliness* to express the pain of being alone. And it has created the word *solitude* to express the glory of being alone."

Make time each day to relax, to be quiet, and to be alone. This is also a good time to practice visualizations and affirmations. I believe it's in spending time alone each day, breathing deeply and quieting our thoughts, that we can do the most for our health, harmony, peacefulness, and living up to our highest potential. Times of quiet, although sometimes hard to create, take a top priority in my life. I devote some time each day, one full day each week, and one three-day weekend each month to solitude and quietude. This regular supplement of silence greatly enhances all areas of my life. As early as I can remember, I have always desired and welcomed spending time in solitude and received great joy in the process. "Every person needs a retreat, a 'dynamo' of silence where he may go for the exclusive purpose of being newly recharged by the Infinite," says Paramahansa Yogananda.

Thoreau has this to say on solitude: "I love to be alone. I never found the companion that was so companionable as solitude." "I have a great deal of company in my house; especially in the morning, when nobody calls." And from Thoreau's *Journal*, March 20, 1841, "It is a great relief when for a few moments in the day we can retire to our chamber to be completely true to ourselves. It leavens the rest of our hours."

Although few of us might choose lifelong solitude, most of us need some time to ourselves. We may differ from our friends, family, and co-workers in the amount and frequency of our need to be alone. We may have a difficult time finding periods of privacy, and even feel guilty claiming them. But when we're deprived of them for too long, we experience distress and a lack of harmony and balance in our lives.

One of my friends has three children. She rarely has time to herself. She is busy running a household, raising the children, and tending the cat, dog, and hamsters. At one point she found herself rushing between the children's dance lessons, doctor appointments, grocery shopping, and other household errands, spending almost no time alone. When she told me how she spent her days,

I became exhausted just listening. I suggested she give herself permission to call some time her own. Now, after she drops off a child at a lesson, she pulls out a favorite book and reads in the car. There are no phones, no people, and no distractions, so she has an hour of quiet and solitude to do or think as she pleases. It's private time, and it's her very own.

Whether it's a few minutes each day or an hour or two, spending some time by yourself is a great rejuvenator. It's like recharging your battery.

I know that sometimes it's hard to find solitude. And sometimes our friends and loved ones don't seem to understand our need to spend some time alone. Anything else will be accepted as okay. We can set aside time for car repairs, office meetings, the gym, or the manicurist. But if we say, "I can't get together with you because that's my time to spend alone," we may be considered antisocial, selfish, rude, or even strange. I urge you to welcome your time alone, even though others may question you. These ideas are expressed beautifully in the book *Gift from the Sea*, by Anne Morrow Lindbergh.

You must make the time to be alone. Make some privacy a priority in your life. Everyone wants some of your time. In order to get quiet time for yourself, reserve a regular time in your daily schedule when the people around you know that, barring emergencies, you expect to be left alone. Explaining your needs clearly and specifically to others will help tremendously.

I enjoy running alone. It's time for myself, for seeing the nature around me, for thinking, and for just letting ideas and visions flow through me. As Emerson has taught me, it's a time when I get out of the way of my divine circuits, just letting the energy flow freely. And so I feel good not only because I'm exercising, but because I'm alone; and there's pleasure and peace in my own company.

So why don't you start today and set aside some time to be still, be quiet, and breathe deeply. If your schedule is really busy, you might consider getting up a little earlier in the morning to fit it in. If you say that your schedule is even too busy for that, I suggest you consider taking a good look at your schedule and simplifying it. If you do, you'll discover, as I have, that "silence is golden" and that it is a wonderful rejuvenator.

You might want to use your time alone to meditate. Meditation is easy and must be experienced on a regular schedule to achieve results. Once a day is helpful, twice a day is recommended, and each session should last fifteen to twenty minutes. (I recommend reading *Autobiography of a Yogi*, and *Divine Romance*, by Paramahansa Yogananda, *Meditation*, by Eknath Easwaran, *An Easy Guide to Meditation*, by Roy Eugene Davis, and *Meditation* magazine for further information.)

I have had a few wonderful teachers of meditation and spiritual understanding, and I would like to acknowledge them here. They include foremost Jesus Christ and Paramahansa Yogananda. Others are *A Course in Miracles*, Roy Eugene Davis, Eknath Easwaran, John R. Price, Dr. Ernest Holmes, Charles Fillmore, Dr. Masaharu Taniguchi, Ralph Waldo Emerson, Eric Butterworth, Emmet Fox, and Dennis Weaver.

The following meditation technique has proven to be useful in lowering blood pressure, reducing stress in the body, clearing the mental field, and calming the emotions. It's a compilation from some of the above great teachers.

1. *In a quiet environment, indoors or outdoors, sit upright, spine straight, and be relaxed. Turn your attention inward, directing your inner gaze either to the space between your eyebrows or to your heart. You might also want to play some peaceful, relaxing music. I sometimes listen to the music of Steven Halpern, who has a variety of tapes and albums. (He also authored an excellent book entitled* Sound Health: The Music and Sounds That Make Us Whole.*)*

2. *As you do this, breathe slowly and deeply. Feel your body breathe air in and out. Do not attempt to regulate the rhythm; just let it flow. Breathe naturally with your diaphragm. Your breath is life itself, but I've noticed that most people don't breathe properly. Watch a baby or a dog breathe when it is still and quiet. It breathes deeply from the abdomen, allowing the air to reach the lower portion of the lungs. Most of us breathe shallowly, shoulders rising, using only the upper portion of the lungs. When we do this, we prevent total relaxation and thereby make it difficult to get in touch with our feeling, intuitive self. Deep breathing goes along with letting go and living fully.*

Start this moment to breathe more deeply as much as possible. To help me in this effort, for a period of six months, I set my watch so that each hour it would beep to remind me to breathe deeply. It took lots of my attention, but after a few months I now quite naturally breathe deeply. I also discover that when I don't, I feel tired. Deep breathing oxygenates the system, increases energy, purifies the blood, cleanses the lymph system, and even improves immune functioning. A study recently completed by Dr. Jack Shields, a lymphologist from Santa Barbara, California, looked at the immune system and its functioning. Dr. Shields put cameras inside people's bodies to see what stimulated cleansing of the lymph system. He found that deep, diaphragmatic breathing is the most effective way to accomplish this. This study reported that deep breathing creates a vacuumlike environment that sucks lymph through the bloodstream and multiplies the pace at which the body eliminates toxins. In fact, deep breathing and exercise can accelerate this process by as much as fifteen times, thereby enhancing the immune system. (For interesting reading, I recommend the book Science of Breath *by* Swami Rama, Rudolph Ballentine, M.D. and Alan Hymes, M.D.)*

So incorporate deep breathing not only into your meditation sessions, but also into your entire day.

3. *If you like, when you breathe in, mentally recite, "I am." When you breathe out, mentally recite a word or phrase that feels good to you, such as "peace," "love," "joy," "I let go and let God," or you might prefer to recite Silent Unity's Prayer for Protection, which goes like this:*

The light of God surrounds me;
The love of God enfolds me;
The power of God protects me;
The presence of God watches over me;
Wherever I am, God is.

Say it at least three times, slowly and deliberately feeling each word. No great effort is required. You might also choose to say your favorite spiritual poem during this initial time.

One of my favorites is the following, by Saint Francis of Assisi:

> Lord, make me an instrument of thy peace.
> Where there is hatred, let me sow love;
> Where there is injury, pardon;
> Where there is doubt, faith;
> Where there is despair, hope;
> Where there is darkness, light;
> Where there is sadness, joy.
>
> Oh Divine Master, grant that I
> May not so much seek
> To be consoled as to console,
> To be understood as to understand,
> To be loved as to love;
> For it is in giving that we receive;
> It is in pardoning that we are pardoned;
> It is in dying (to self) that
> We are born to eternal life.

Whatever you do say, it should be meaningful to you; memorize it so you can keep your eyes closed. I also like to end my meditation with the affirmation, "I choose to spend this day in perfect peace."

4. *For those of you who want to meditate more deeply, try the following. After you are deeply relaxed, continue to explore the inner spaces of your consciousness. Listen and look within. If you hear an inner sound, dissolve in the sound and gently be willing to seek out the origin of the sound. If you perceive an inner light, proceed with it the same as with the inner sound. If you hear a voice, just be still and listen. Move through all that is perceived, whether sound, light, or voice, until you experience a feeling of lighter consciousness. Rest for as long as you can in the experience.*

5. *After experiencing deep rest, mental calm, and perhaps a sense of pure awareness (this doesn't happen every time, especially if you are a beginner), you will naturally experience an outflow of attention, bringing your meditation to a close. (If you have a limited amount of time, keep a clock nearby.)*

6. *While resting in the calm of meditation, be appreciative of life, and bless yourself as lovely, capable, and lovable. Bless others with whom you share your life. Bless humanity and the world with love and recognition.*

7. *While resting in this meditative mood, if you wish you may also do the following: Think about the meaning of life; who you really are; your purpose or mission. Think without limit. When the mental field is clear and the emotional nature calm, this is a good time to visualize your goals, seeing them with perfect results. With creative imagination, feel the emotions of joy and thanksgiving as if this were your current reality. Conclude with visualizing world peace.*

8. *Then gently go about your day's schedule. Do not be anxious for results. Just practice regularly and be patient. In a short time you will notice positive changes: inner calm and attunement with the world.*

Yes, solitude fosters peace and enables you to get in touch with the great love and light within. Through spending time alone you realize you are never alone. This certainty is real peace, true serenity. I also believe that it's from spending time in solitude that we learn to live more from inner guidance, rather than externally. Too often people look outside themselves for happiness and fulfillment. Nothing will ever be enough until you are enough, and when you are enough, then anything will be enough.

Some of the most heartwarming realizations I have come to through meditation are that I am already free, I am more than I could ever imagine, and that I can simply be happy and whole because that's already my divine nature. This is said so aptly in the fascinating and lovely book *Way of the Peaceful Warrior,* by Dan Millman.

Wake up, wake up! Soon the person you believe you are will die—so now, wake up and be content with this knowledge: There is no need to search; achievement leads to nowhere. It makes no difference at all, so just be happy now. Love is the only reality of the world, because it is all One, you see. And the only laws are paradox, humor, and change. There is no problem, never was, and never will be. Release your struggle, let go of your mind, throw away your concerns, and relax into the world. No need to resist life; just do your best. Open your eyes and see that you are far more than you imagine. You are the world, you are the universe; you are yourself and everyone else, too. It's all the marvelous Play of God. Wake up, regain your humor. Don't worry, just be happy. You are already free.

With the realization that you are already enough, that you are the gift, and that you can live from inner guidance, your life will be immensely enriched. And in turn, your life will enrich the quality of life on this planet. Living from internal awareness brings a deep sense of peace and security. You do not need to search for approval or recognition from the outer, for you carry love's approval and recognition within. You glow with a radiance, and life takes on new meaning and purpose. You live thankfully and wear a smile of joy and contentment. You embrace life. You love living. *Your love for life always brings out the best in you.*

Let go of and avoid those things that interfere with your inner peace. The result: wisdom. Wisdom is a natural part of finding peace and happiness within yourself through thoughts and actions that are in harmony with your real Self. But this necessitates governing your mind wisely, with discernment, by dwelling on the positive aspects of life. Be circumspect in all your actions. Resolve to develop your spiritual powers more earnestly from this day forward.

If you have joy, you have everything. So learn the art of living joyfully, and be glad and contented. Laugh at yourself and the world. Have and *be* happiness now. All it takes is your willing acceptance of it.

One of my favorite books is *Gifts From Eykis*, by Dr.Wayne Dyer. A delightful and insightful book, it is a parable for our time. A woman from another planet comes to Earth and imparts wisdom and simple truths to apply to our own lives, and to the healing of our planet. Throughout the book is one recurring thought, which touches a responsive chord in me: *There is no way to happiness; happiness is the way.*

As we become healthier and happier, as we increasingly radiate goodness and positiveness, we help to make our world more harmonious in every way. We have a responsibility to ourselves and to humanity to live fully—healthfully, joyfully, and peacefully. Some may think this selfish. But when you enjoy living and are enthusiastic about life, you are never a burden to anyone, and that's the most unselfish thing you can do. Enthusiasm comes from the Greek word *entheos*, and means "to be filled with God." So as you let your light shine, and live filled with enthusiasm for this gift of life, you inspire others to live fully. That's unselfishness.

Living enthusiastically will help you know and appreciate the wonder of life. I marvel at the simple yet intricate web of life that supports and sustains us. The song of life sings through all of us (the uni-verse) fully and freely. Be happy to be alive. Celebrate your beingness and our oneness.

Understand that on one level we are all the same, are all one. My dear friend, Rev. George Marks, assistant minister of Founders Church in Los Angeles, reminds me "The Spirit of All Life seeks expression through those individuals who, through Divine Love, open their hearts to one another and reflect the Light so all may live together in peace." When we live from the heart, we realize that together we can do so much. Look at the wonderful results of the efforts of the musicians who have come together to raise money to end world hunger.

Look for ways you can be of service. When helping others you quickly forget your small self and you feel and know your larger Self. As the illuminating rays of the sun nurture, so should you strive to let your light shine. Try to spread rays of hope to those without hope, foster courage in those who have given up, and rekindle the light of strength in those who believe they are failures. As we reach out and touch one another, the planet is made lighter.

I am reminded of a terrific movie I've seen several times, *Oh, God.* In it George Burns plays God and John Denver plays Jerry

Landers. One scene in particular moved me. It takes place in Landers's bathroom when he first comes face to face with God. Landers asks God why he chose this time to appear. God says that he made the world to work, but he looks down now and we are filling his rivers with waste, we are polluting his air; we're wasting his world. When Landers asks God why he doesn't do something about it God says that humanity should do something about it. Landers replies that humanity needs help. And to that, God replies, *"That's why I gave you each other."*

I was moved by the truth in this exchange. We are here on Earth for each other, not against each other. We are here to learn about love and to grow from love. We are here not to see through each other but to see each other through. This world was made to work. We have everything that it takes for our world to grow harmoniously and fruitfully, to be fulfilling and joyous for every human being and living creature. But it is only when we all start acting with these truths in mind that we will make the world work.

As a way of joining together toward our common goal of world peace, I suggest the following: every day plan to spend a minimum of one minute in quiet meditation or contemplation of peace, beginning at exactly noon (EST), 11:00 A.M. (CST), 10:00 A.M. (MST), or 9:00 A.M. (PST). (Those of you in different parts of the world, adjust your time accordingly.) During this time visualize, affirm, and be thankful for world peace—an idea whose time is now. Relax and mentally align with and feel the energy of millions joining with you in imagining a peaceful, radiant, loving planet Earth. Make your vision vivid. Willingly let your inner guidance show you what to do. Be appreciative of world peace.

If this specific time doesn't work well for you, or if you miss it, or if you want to do it twice, every day at noon your time, devote at least one minute to another joint meditation on world peace. (Because there is really no separate time in space, all over the world we will be simultaneously focusing on our common goal. We will be making a difference.)

Peace in the world has never been more important than it is right now. We all agree that peace is an idea whose time has come. Yet we often make peace in our personal lives conditional on another person's actions or reactions, and peace in the world conditional on another nation's actions or reactions. *The only real condition essential for peace is our commitment to it and our acceptance of it.* Let all of you who are reading this today say "Yes" to world peace.

You make a difference in the world. Since your birth you have touched countless lives. If you weren't here the tapestry of life would be incomplete and lacking. This idea is poignantly expressed in the 1947 movie classic by Frank Capra, *It's a Wonderful Life.* In the movie Jimmy Stewart gets to see how his town would have been sadly different if he had not lived. Live in gratitude and peace.

Victor Hugo said, "Nothing is more powerful than an idea whose time has come." I would add that there is also nothing more powerful than an idea to which we collectively direct our inner light and strength. Clearly, individually we can do much toward making this world a peaceful home for everyone.

You may be saying, "Now how can I alone really make any difference at all?" Well, let's take a look at one perfect example. Would you think that an eleven-year-old schoolgirl from Manchester, Maine, could make a difference in world peace? Well, that's exactly what Samantha Smith did. The world is a better place because this girl cared, had an idea, and summoned the courage to go after what she believed in. PBS presented a tribute to Samantha Smith entitled "Peace Child." In addition to highlighting Samantha's trip to Russia, there was a live satellite connection between Minneapolis and Moscow, in which a group of children from each city had an opportunity to talk with each other. There was also a wonderful duet sung by an American girl and a Russian boy. As I sit here I get teary-eyed just thinking about that duet, and the impact of one child who followed her heart and taught us that one person can indeed make a difference.

Two very special doctors are also making a difference. The friendship and collaboration of these two men is one of the small miracles of our lifetime. American Bernard Lown and Russian Yevgeny Chazov, both leading heart specialists, transcended Cold War politics to found the International Physicians for the Prevention of Nuclear War (IPPNW). They have been awarded the Nobel peace prize for their efforts.

In December 1980 Lown, Chazov, and four colleagues met in Geneva to work out the principles of the IPPNW. The following year they met near Washington, D.C., and have continued to meet regularly to address letters to Soviet and American leaders and to publish papers on the medical consequences of nuclear war. Chazov says there are four million doctors in the world, and he hopes to recruit at least half of them. The group's members have no special expertise in solving international conflicts, but their medical training gives them a keen awareness of the consequences of failing to do so. They know that the medical profession cannot handle a disaster on the scale of a nuclear war.

> Controlled, universal disarmament is the imperative for our time. The demand for it by the hundreds of millions will, I hope, become so universal and so insistent that no man, no government anywhere, can withstand it.
>
> —Dwight D. Eisenhower

Robert Muller, Ph.D., is another person making a difference. Dr. Muller, a citizen of France and doctor of law and economics, has been serving in the United Nations since 1948. He is a former assistant secretary-general of the United Nations, and most recently served as the organizer for the United Nations anniversary celebration. He is now the chancellor of the University of Peace, headquartered in Costa Rica, which is an international postgraduate institution chartered by the United Nations. The guiding principle is unity in diversity, and the focus is on the emerging interdependent global society. (See the resource directory for more information.)

Dag Hammarskjöld, who also filled the role of U.N. secretary-general, and whom Muller called "one of the great mystics of our time, who showed the world that the way to sanctity passes through the world of action," inspired Muller to begin his spiritual journey. His friendship with U Thant, a Buddhist and U.N. secretary-general following Hammarskjöld's death, called "a master of the art of living," changed Dr. Muller's life. Muller came to believe that at this time, our greatest need is for masters who present good examples. Like U Thant, they ought to include people in high public office and with wide ranges of reponsibility. *Most of All They Taught Me Happiness*, Muller's first book, offers us hope and solutions for these challenging times. In his two latest books, *What War Taught Me About Peace* and *The Birth of a Global Civilization*, he shows how even in the face of potentially devastating problems our human spirit remains steadfastly strong and joyful.

> *Decide to be peaceful*
> *Render others peaceful*
> *Be a model of peace*
> *Irradiate your peace*
> *Love passionately the peace*
>   *of our beautiful planet*
> *Do not listen to the warmongers,*
>   *hateseeders and powerseekers*
> *Dream always of a peaceful,*
>   *warless, disarmed world*
> *Think always of a peaceful world*
> *Work always for a peaceful world*
> *Switch on and keep on, in yourself,*
>   *the peaceful buttons,*
>   *those marked love,*
>   *serenity, happiness, truth,*
>   *kindness, friendliness,*
>   *understanding and tolerance*
> *Pray and thank God every day for peace*
> *Pray for the United Nations*
>   *and all peacemakers*
> *Pray for the leaders of nations*
>   *who hold the peace of the world*
>   *in their hands*
> *Pray God to let our planet at long last*
>   *become the Planet of Peace*

And sing in unison with all humanity:
"Let there be peace on Earth
And let it begin with me."

—Robert Muller

Dr. Muller updates the prediction of Teilhard de Chardin, the Jesuit paleontologist, who said "world harmony would be achieved in the human race in 5,000 years," by giving us suggestions for how world peace can be reached by the year 2010.

Last week, I had a beautiful dream. Our country selected two children-ambassadors (a girl and a boy) from each state to go to Russia and live for a year as foreign exchange students. Likewise, we lovingly received one hundred students from Russia to our country. We got to see that no matter what country we're from, we're really all the same in our hearts. I do believe that the children know this better than anyone, and if we're to create a world of peace and harmony, we must listen to the children and heed their guidance and advice.

I would like to take this opportunity to talk about another urgent issue of our time—ending world hunger. Are you aware that thirty-five thousand people die each day as a consequence of hunger—twenty-four people every minute? In study after study, prestigious international commissions have come to one conclusion: humanity now possesses the resources and technology to end hunger by the end of this century. What it will take is a worldwide commitment to get the job done.

The Hunger Project is dedicated to getting that job done. To date more that 3.4 million individuals living in 152 countries have enrolled in The Hunger Project as a powerful, personal expression of a commitment to eliminating hunger once and for all. To write the organization for more information, see the resource directory for the address. I also recommend that you read The Hunger Project book, *Ending Hunger: An Idea Whose Time Has Come.*

Another organization dedicated to ending world hunger is The End Hunger Network. It is a nonprofit organization representing an alliance of more than 130 private and voluntary organizations, media professionals, corporations, government agencies, community groups, and individuals working collectively toward the goal of ending world hunger and creating world peace. The End Hunger Network communicates the shared goals of its members through the mass media, producing events and educational programs to generate public awareness, understanding, support for, and involvement in the campaign to end hunger.

LIFE is yet another organization that helps feed the hungry. An acronym for Love is Feeding Everyone, LIFE was started in 1983 by actors Dennis Weaver and Valerie Harper. It now feeds more than 23,000 people every day of the year. The project runs on a simple idea. Each day food that would normally be discarded is picked up from supermarkets: dated dairy products, deli products, and baked goods, slightly limp produce, and damaged products, such as dented cans. All of these food items are still nutritious, but are not as marketable as the stores like them to be. This food is then taken to a distribution center. There the food is washed if necessary, packaged, and sorted into large orders, which are picked up once a week by different agencies, such as a church, a shelter for battered women, or a drug rehabilitation facility. Sometimes LIFE also services soup kitchens on Skid Row. Currently there are two centers in Los Angeles, and LIFE is working to get others started in that area.

Because what LIFE picks up from the supermarkets doesn't make a totally well-rounded diet, another important part of this successful program is food drives. Volunteers sit at a table outside a supermarket, tell customers about LIFE, and ask the shoppers if they would buy an extra bag of beans, an extra canned item, or perhaps an extra bottle of oil to drop off on their way out.

LIFE volunteers would like to pass on to other communities what they have learned. This program can work any place in the United States where there are willing, committed people and supermarkets, because supermarkets always have much waste. With this in mind, LIFE has created a how-to manual and a video film that show people exactly what LIFE does and how those in other cities can get started.

Wouldn't it be wonderful to see LIFE in every major city in this country? You can make it happen. You can make a difference.

Windstar is a nonprofit organization in Colorado co-founded by John Denver and Thomas Crum to create a sustainable future for the planet. The Foundation's director sees Windstar as a tool that can become a "planetary consciousness shifter." A decade ago no one thought the hunger problem could even be solved; today's efforts have proven that notion wrong. They want people to realize that the same transformation can happen in the areas of energy and peace.

Windstar has many impressive programs. It sponsors a variety of educational programs, including children's workshops in music and science, volunteers for peace, international exchanges, Global Games, Aiki with Tom Crum, and other programs geared toward living at one's highest potential. They also offer an excellent annual symposium, hosted by John Denver, called "Choices for the Future." Write and ask to be on Windstar's mailing list; the address is in the resource directory.

> We need not wait for leadership. We can begin to effect change at any point in a complex system: a human life, a family, a nation. One person can create a transformative environment for others through trust and friendship.
>
> —Marilyn Ferguson, *The Aquarian Conspiracy*

What else can we, as individuals, do? We can read books on peace and living fully, such as, *Love is Letting go of Fear,* by Jerry Jampolsky, M.D.; and *Peace Pilgrim,* by Peace Pilgrim. Also, we can read *Celebrate Yourself!,* by Eric Butterworth; *Bible, The Divine Romance,* by Paramahansa Yogananda; *"Only Love,"* by Sri Daya Mata; *You'll See It When You Believe It,* by Dr. Wayne Dyer; or *Chop Wood, Carry Water—A Guide to Finding Spiritual Fulfillment in Everyday Life,* by Rick Fields. We can write our government leaders and vote for those who are making a difference, who are committed to creating a world that works. We can commend those who have done something worthwhile for peace. Also, we can get involved in or even start a community peace fellowship or peace study group. We can attend or sponsor public meetings on the subject of peace. We can also donate our time or money to groups dedicated to promoting peace.

But ultimately peace begins within. The situation in the world is but a reflection of the situation within human beings, a reflection of our awareness. *Peace within ourselves is the first step toward peace in our world.* And the way to inner peace is through love.

Peace starts with you and with everything that you think, feel, and do. In every relationship that you have, show yourself to be a loving, forgiving, compassionate person. Love, forgiveness, compassion first start with and for yourself, and then flow out to your family and friends. Expanding, they encompass all whom you touch—the world of human beings. It is in this way that all inequities will be eventually righted, harmony will prevail, and true peace will be achieved. In other words, by changing ourselves, we change the world.

Dr. Robert Muller invites us to ask ourselves, "How can I be of service to creation?" and then adds, "You cannot expect the world to change, before you change yourself."

Before we can change, *we must make a conscious choice to start doing things differently.* Choose those things that work for you.

Choose to follow your inner light—it will illume your path. Perhaps you'll choose to do things slightly different than your family and friends. That's okay. "If a man does not keep pace with his companions, perhaps it is because he hears a different drummer. Let him step to the music he hears, however measured or far away," said Thoreau. Follow your heart. The more you follow and surrender to your heart, the more you will celebrate the divinity of your essence.

Choose to be open to new ways, new truths. Start reading books, attending workshops, watching videos, and listening to tapes—and asking questions. Experiment with new, healthier ways of eating. Begin being more physically active.

Choose happiness. It's your birthright. When you choose personal peace and happiness, you can be healthy. And remember it's not about arriving, for you have already arrived. *It's about being who you are.* It's about being happy with who and where you are. Health and happiness go hand in hand.

Choose to think beautiful and magnificent thoughts, and beauty and magnificence will be yours. Choose to always think your highest thoughts. When thinking of yourself and others, choose loving thoughts. Your world is the product of your thoughts. Through patient practice you can learn to adjust your mental attitude, at will, to create your own miracles. If you wander off course, and we all do once in awhile, a moment of quiet lovingness will get you centered again. You'll be balanced and ready to experience, once again, the celebration of life.

Choose to embrace life by committing yourself to a wellness program. As you choose to move forward in the direction of your dreams and begin to live the life you have imagined, you will be radiantly alive and healthy. Choose to celebrate life and live fully—healthfully, joyfully, and peacefully. Together we will create a New World—a kingdom of light, love, peace, forgiveness, health, joy, and understanding.

I salute you and support you in your great adventure.

Peace,

—Susan Smith Jones

Self-Discovery Questions

1. *What do I want most out of life?*

2. *What is my personal definition of success?*

3. *When I feel negative emotions, do I usually blame someone else?*

4. *When do I feel most happy and at peace? Does it originate outside me or within me?*

5. *How do I feel about being alone?*

6. *What are things I do to avoid being alone and having quietude?*

7. *How old do I feel?*

8. *What changes can I make in my attitude that will enrich my life?*

9. *If I knew I had only one year to live, what changes would I make in my life? Why aren't I making those changes now?*

10. *What does peace mean to me?*

Action Choices

1. *This is the time during each day that I have set aside just for me:*

2. *Following are ways I choose to simplify my life:*

3. *In the past, my negative emotions have sometimes immobilized me. This is ending because I now choose to do the following instead:*

4. *Following are at least ten things I love about myself and my world:*

5. *Here is a list of affirmations that support my magnificence:*

6. *If this were the last year of my life, the following things would be most important to me:*

7. *These are some changes I can make in my life to experience more peace:*

8. Here are some things I am going to do to enrich life on this planet:

Namaste*

*A Sanskrit word meaning "I salute the light within you."

PEACE IN THE WORLD

When there is wellness in the mind,
There will be wholeness in the person.

When there is wholeness in the person,
There will be harmony in the home.

When there is harmony in the home,
There will be forgiveness in the nation.

When there is forgiveness in the nation,
There will be peace in the world.

—Susan Smith Jones

Target Exercise Heart Rate*

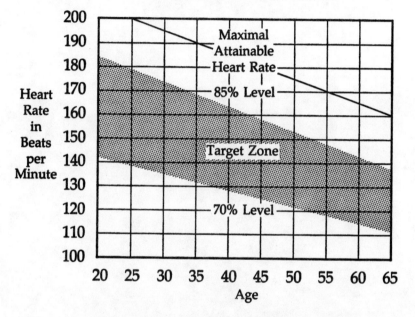

*According to the principles of exercise programming set forth by the American Heart Association and the President's Council on Physical Fitness.

RESOURCE
DIRECTORY

ALL-1
Nutritech
719 Haley Street
Santa Barbara, CA 93103
(800) 235-5727 (in CA - (805) 963-9581)

ALL-1 is a pure nutrient powder. Mixed with your favorite juice, it provides over 50 vitamins, minerals and amino acids. For more information or a free sample contact Nutritech.

AMERICAN NATURAL HYGIENE SOCIETY
Health Science magazine
P.O. Box 30630
Tampa, FL 33630

This wonderful organization publishes the award-winning *Health Science* magazine. Annual membership dues are $25.00, which includes a subscription to *Health Science*. Members also receive discounts on books, seminars, lectures, etc. Write to the above address and become a member.

AMERICAN OCEANS CAMPAIGN
2219 Main Street, Suite 2B
Santa Monica, CA 90405
(213) 452-2206

Started by actor Ted Danson, AOC is dedicated to the restoration and preservation of the ocean environment. To receive a newsletter, contact above.

A.R.E. (Association for Research and Enlightenment, Inc.)
P.O. Box 595
Virginia Beach, VA 23451
(804) 428-3588

For more information on Edgar Cayce's work, or to be on their mailing list, contact above.

BERNARD JENSEN INTERNATIONAL
Route 1, Box 52
Escondido, CA 92025
(619) 749-2727

For more information on all his books, including *Chlorella: Gem of the Orient*, cassettes and study program, write to the above address.

BODYSLANT and **BODY LIFT**
P.O. Box 1667-S
Newport Beach, CA 92663
(800) 443-3917, ext. 202

The BodySlant is a superb slant board which also functions as a bed and ottoman. I recommend using it daily. The Body Lift is a simple, comfortable way to stand your body upside down so your shoulders rest on a thick cushion, your head dangles off the floor, and your neck stretches naturally. I've used both my BodySlant and Body Lift for over 15 years and recommend them highly.

BUCKMINSTER FULLER INSTITUTE
1743 South La Cienega Boulevard
Los Angeles, CA 90035
(213) 837-7710

Disseminates information on Fuller's work and ideas.

CAL-a-VIE
2249 Somerset Road
Vista, CA 92084
(619) 945-2055

An excellent spa for fostering high-level awareness. Cal-a-Vie is my favorite spa which I visit at least once a year. It offers the ambience, fitness programs, health and beauty treatments to rejuvenate the whole body, mind and spirit. Nutritionist Yvonne Nienstadt and Chef Rosie provide an exceptional nutrition education and superlative cuisine.

CELEBRATE LIFE!
Audiocassette series by Susan Smith Jones, Ph.D.
Includes seven tapes:

1a. "The Main Ingredients: Positive Thinking & the Mind"
1b. "The Main Ingredients: Exercise, Nutrition & Relaxation"
2a. "Get High on Life Through Exercise"
2b. "Make Your Exercise Program a Great Adventure"
3a. "Nutrition for Aliveness"
3b. "Superlative Dining"
4a. "Your Thoughts May Be Fattening"
4b. "Living Lightly, Naturally Trim"
5a. "Experience Aliveness"
5b. "Learn From Children How To Celebrate Life"
6a. "The Joy of Solitude & The Art of Serenity"
6b. "Relaxation & Meditation: Natural & Easy"
7a. "Celebrate Your Magnificence"
7b. "Affirm a Beautiful Life"

To order the entire seven-tape package, send $75.00 (or $12.50 per tape), U.S. check or money order only, payable to: Health Unlimited, P.O. Box 49396, Los Angeles, CA 90049.

For more information on the tapes, send a business size, stamped, self-addressed envelope to the above address.

CENTER FOR SCIENCE IN THE PUBLIC INTEREST
Executive Director - Dr. Michael Jacobson
1501 16th Street N.W.
Washington, D.C. 20036

Write for their literature on nutrition and their excellent Nutrition Action Newsletter.

CENTER FOR SPIRITUAL AWARENESS
Roy Eugene Davis
P.O. Box 7, Lake Rabun Road
Lakemont, GA 30552
(404) 782-4723

To find out about the retreat center, the *Truth Journal,* and a variety of spiritual books and related material, write to the above.

A COURSE IN MIRACLES
Foundation for Inner Peace
P.O. Box 635
Tiburon, CA 94920

DE ANGELIS, DR. BARBARA
1904 Centinela Avenue
Los Angeles, CA 90025
(213) 820-6600

For information on Dr. De Angelis's *Making Love Work* seminars, her workshops or conferences, contact the office above.

✳ DIAMOND ORGANICS
P.O. Box 2159
Freedom, CA 95019
(800) 922-2396

For several years, Diamond Organics has been providing high quality fresh organic produce to chefs at the finest restaurants and hotels. Their produce is now available to individuals and can be shipped directly to your home or office. They carry all types of organic produce including specialty greens and lettuce, citrus fruits, vegetables, roots, tubers, sprouts, etc. No minimum order is required. I order from this superb company regularly. Call or write for a brochure.

EARTHSAVE
706 Frederick Street
Santa Cruz, CA 95062-2205
(408) 423-4069

Founded by John Robbins, author of a *Diet for a New America*, EarthSave is a nonprofit organization providing education and leadership for transition to more healthful and environmentally sound food choices, non-polluting energy supplies and a wiser use of natural resources. For more information and free literature, write or call.

EARTHTRUST
2500 Pali Highway
Honolulu, HI 96817
(808) 595-6927

Have you ever wanted to adopt a whale? Now is your chance. Originally formed in 1976 as "Save the Whales," the organization has since changed its name to "Earthtrust" and presently works to protect a wide variety of endangered species and preserve our planet's natural environment. Write for more information on how you can participate.

FRIENDS OF THE UNIVERSITY OF PEACE FOUNDATION
P.O. Box 20461
New York, NY 10011

GREENPEACE
1436 U Street, N.W.
P.O. Box 3720
Washington, D.C. 20007
(202) 462 1177

HEAL THE BAY
1640 5th Street
Santa Monica, CA 90401
(800) HEALBAY

A nonprofit coalition of people and organizations committed to restoring and maintaining the chemical, physical, and biological integrity of the nation's waters. To receive a newsletter or more information, call them.

"HOW TO ACHIEVE ANY GOAL: THE MAGIC OF CREATIVE VISUALIZATION/LIVING YOUR VISION/COMMITMENT"
A one and a half hour audiocassette by Susan Smith Jones. Includes a twenty-minute meditation you can use every day to help you realize your goals and dreams. To order, please send $12.50, U.S. money order or check only, payable to: Health Unlimited, P.O. Box 49396, Los Angeles, CA 90049.

JONES, SUSAN SMITH
Lectures, seminars, and workshops for your organization. For information regarding booking a presentation or consultation, contact Health Unlimited, P.O. Box 49396, Los Angeles, CA 90049, Attn: Director.

JUICEMAN JUICER
JM Marketing
655 South Orcas, Suite 22D
Seattle, WA 98108
(800) 800-8455 (to inquire about the purchase of products)
(206) 762-8405 (for customer service)

The Juiceman Juicer is an excellent juicer which I use regularly. To receive their newsletter, catalog of books and products, or for more information, contact above.

KEN KEYES CENTER
790 Commercial Avenue
Coos Bay, OR 97420
(503) 267-6412

For a free catalog of workshops, send your name and address to the Registrar. You will receive a quarterly catalog listing excellent nonprofit workshops, books, and audio and video tapes. I also give several workshops at the Center.

 KYOLIC
Wakunaga of America Co., Ltd.
23501 Madero
Mission Viejo, CA 92691
(800) 421-2998 (except CA)
(800) 544-5800 (in CA)

This company offers Kyo-Green, a nutritious drink made from a unique blend of young barley, wheat grass, kelp, brown rice, and chlorella. For a free trial pack of Kyo-Green, call above.

LIFE
Love Is Feeding Everyone
310 North Fairfax, Second Floor
Los Angeles, CA 90036
(213) 936-0895

LIFETIME STAINLESS STEEL CORPORATION
c/o Mr. Stephen Foti, President
12 Railroad Street
Fishers, NY 14453

Write for their full-color brochure of their cooking utensils.

NATIONAL WILDLIFE FEDERATION
1412 16th Street, N.W.
Washington, D.C. 20036
(202) 637-3700

To encourage the intelligent management of the life-sustaining resources of the earth and promote a greater appreciation of their resources, their community relationship, and wise use.

NATURE'S WAY PRODUCTS, INC.
Efamol Evening Primrose Oil
Liquid Chlorophyll
Primadophilus
10 Mountain Springs Parkway
Springville, UT 84663
1-800-453-1468

NEW BALANCE ATHLETIC SHOES
38-42 Everett Street
Boston, MA 02134
(617) 783-4000

NIGHTINGALE-CONANT CORPORATION
7300 North Lehigh Avenue
Chicago, IL 60610
(800) 323-3938

Offers a wide variety of audiocassettes on living fully.

OCEAN KAYAK, INC.
(800) 852-9257

Ocean Kayak originated the sit-on-top kayak in 1971. This design is excellent for the beginner as well as the advanced paddler. Kayaking is one of my favorite ways to exercise. Call for more information.

PAWLING HEALTH MANOR
Director—Joy Gross
Box 401
Hyde Park, N.Y. 12538
(914) 889-4141

Offers a rejuvenating holistic program which includes vegetarian foods and surpervised fasting.

PEACE PILGRIM
Friends of Peace Pilgrim
43480 Cedar Avenue
Hemet, CA 92544
(714) 927-7678

To receive a free 32-page booklet, *Steps Toward Inner Peace*, the 200 page *Peace Pilgrim*, and an inspiring newsletter, write to the above address. Friends of Peace Pilgrim is a non-profit, tax-exempt, all volunteer organization. Donations are welcomed, but not required.

PERFECT 7
Agape Health Products
4431 Corporate Center Drive
Los Alamito, CA 90720
(714) 229-8866
(800) 767-4776

Perfect 7 is an excellent psyllium-based herbal poweder (mix with water or juice), used to encourage healthy bowel management and detoxification. Write or call for more information.

POWERBAR
1442 A Walnut Street
Berkeley, CA 94709
(800) 444-5154

The PowerBar is a delicious sustained-energy bar for endurance athletes and active people. It combines healthful ingredients and important nutrients. It's also low in fat. PowerBars are an essential part of my training program. For more information or a free newsletter, call the above number.

PRECOR USA
P.O. Box 3004
Bothell, WA 98041-3004
(800) 4-PRECOR

For more information on PRECOR's excellent high-end home fitness equipment, call or write.

PRINCE OF PEACE ENTERPRISES, INC.
3450 Third Street, Suite 3-G
San Francisco, CA 94124
(800) 52-PEACE

This excellent company has the exclusive distributorship of the vitamin supplement Bio-Strath and other health care products. For a copy of their brochure, write or call.

QUARTUS FOUNDATION FOR SPIRITUAL RESEARCH
John R. Price
P.O. Box 1768
Boerne, TX 78006-6768
(512) 537-4689

Write for the Quartus introductory packet which includes information on John Price's books and tapes.

SCIENCE OF MIND MAGAZINE
P.O. Box 75127
Los Angeles, CA 90075
(213) 388-2181

Inspiring reading. Published monthly for $18.00 per year.

SEA & EARTH HEALTH PRODUCTS
P.O. Box 330-A
Mamaroneck, NY 10543
(800) 431-2582

Mail order company offering a variety of well-known health products and supplements.

SELF-REALIZATION FELLOWSHIP
3880 San Rafael Avenue
Los Angeles, CA 90065

Write for information on Paramahansa Yogananda, books, and Self-Realization Fellowship centers.

SIERRA CLUB
730 Polk Street
San Francisco, CA 94109
(415) 776-2211

The Sierra Club exists to explore, enjoy and protect all wilderness on our planet. Become a member and help protect our environment.

SIMONTON CANCER CENTER
875 Via de La Paz
Pacific Palisades, CA 90272

SEICHO-NO-IE
14527 South Vermont Avenue
Gardena, CA 90247
(213) 323-8486

Write for more information on Dr. Masaharu Taniguchi and his Truth of Life Movement and his publications.

SOUND RX
P.O. Box 151439
San Rafael, CA 94915
(800) 726-9243 (outside CA)
(800) 453-9800 (inside CA)

To receive a catalog of Steven Halpern's music, call or write.

TAYLOR'S HERB GARDERN
1535 Lone Oak Road
Vista, CA 92084
(619) 727-3485

Taylor's Herb Garden offers a variety of herbs for seasoning and gardens in both plant and seed form. You can have them delivered right to yyour door. Call or write for their beautiful color brochure.

TREE OF LIFE SEMINARS
Gabriel Cousens, M.D.
200 Spring Hill Road
Petaluma, CA 94952
(707) 778-6501 (8:00-8:30 a.m. or 1:00-2:00 p.m., Tuesday through Thursday)

Dr. Cousens offers a variety of excellent seminars and retreats on nutrition and your spiritual life, rejuvenation, fasting, Reiki training, Hatha Yoga, etc. Call or write to receive more information.

TREK USA
801 W. Madison Street
Waterloo, WI 53594
(414) 478-2191

Trek makes mountain and road bikes of the highest quality. For more information, check with your local bicycle dealer or write Trek directly.

UNITY MAGAZINE & RETREAT CENTER
Unity School of Christianity
Unity Village, MO 64065

Write for information on their lovely retreat village which offers workshops and classes.

UNIVERSAL GYM EQUIPMENT
930 27th Avenue S.W.
Cedar Rapids, IA 52406
(800) 553-7901

Write for a full-color brochure on their gym equipment.

VOLVIC
Great Waters of France, Inc.
Volvic Marketing Department
777 Putnam Avenue
Greenwich, CT 06830

For more information on this pure, delicious water, write to the above address.

WESTBRAE NATURAL FOODS
P.O. Box 8711
Emeryville, CA 94602
(415) 658-7521

Write for more information on their Brown Rice Syrup (organic and traditional) as well as their other health promoting food products.

THE WINDSTAR FOUNDATION
P.O. Box 286
Snowmass, CO 81654
(303) 927-4777

WORLD HAPPINESS AND COOPERATION
P.O. Box 1153
Anacortes, WA 98221

Exclusively sells the work of Robert Muller. Write for a listing of his books.

A F T E R W O R D

*"Let your example change others' Lives.
Reform yourself and you will reform thousands."*

—Paramahansa Yogananda

The choices we select in life clearly determine the quality of our lives. With consciousness about who and what we are, and with a commitment to ourselves and to each other, we can make life work for everyone on this planet. For just a moment, close your eyes and see the planet in your mind's eye, viewing it from outer space as the astronauts have seen it. Notice the land masses and oceans without man-made boundaries or borders. See our earthly home in resplendent hues of green, aqua, blue, and white—magnificence overflowing with natural resources to supply everyone's needs.

Now take a closer look. Focus on the people who inhabit our planet. Look past nationality or race, and recognize that we as the human family are overwhelmingly more alike than we are different. Notice both the shared humanity and spirituality of all human beings and of all creation. Now look closer into the hearts of all beings and see the great depths of compassion and caring, people who love their families and neighbors, people whose goals are peace and harmony for all.

All life is interconnected. We are all one—and as we choose to be healthy and live heart-to-heart, person-to-person, in cooperation, the quality of life on our planet will be transformed. We are all members of a glorious global family. As we let go of the illusion of separation, and as we awaken and commit to being radiantly healthy and fully alive, we will recognize the profound oneness of all Life. Then by acting from this awareness and linking with other members of our family, we will create a living system that sharply accelerates the peaceful transformation of our planet.

Make a conscious choice to give of yourself today and everyday. It was Ralph Waldo Emerson who once said, "The only gift is a portion of thyself." I believe that it first starts in the hearts of each one of us. We have choices to make as to how we want to live and how we want our world to be. Health is a conscious choice. Peace is a conscious choice. Forgiveness is a conscious choice.

When we reach out to another and offer unconditional love and forgiveness, joy and peace are the result. We can enrich the quality of life on our planet and we can, together, create a world where everyone wins. Don't feel that you are powerless or insignificant in affecting a change in what appears to be "overwhelming" obstacles or major crises on our planet. Everything you do or feel or think or say makes a difference. Every action you take is contributing to the whole. And just perhaps, you will be the one our world has been waiting for.

From *New Fables (Thus Spoke the Caribou)* by Kurt Kauter, (out of print) is this lovely story:

"Tell me the weight of a snowflake," a coalmouse (a small bird) asked a wild dove.

"Nothing more than nothing," was the answer.

"In that case, I must tell you a marvelous story," the coalmouse said.

"I sat on the branch of a fir, close to its trunk, when it began to snow—not heavily, not a raging blizzard—no, just like a dream, without wind, without any violence. Since I did not have anything better to do, I counted the snowflakes settling on the twigs and needles of my branch. Their number was exactly 3,741,952. When the 3,741,953rd dropped onto the branch, nothing more than nothing as you say, the branch broke off." Having said that, the coalmouse flew away. The dove, since Noah's time an authority on the matter, thought about the story for awhile, and finally said to herself, "Perhaps there is only one person's voice lacking for peace to come to the world."

Embrace life. Live fully. And extend your blessings of love, appreciation, forgiveness, and oneness to every person in our world.

—Susan Smith Jones

ABOUT THE AUTHOR

Susan Smith Jones, B.A. (Psychology), Teaching Credential, M.S. (Kinesiology), Ph.D. (Health Sciences) has been a fitness instructor to students, staff, and faculty at UCLA for the past 20 years. As a freelance writer, her more than 500 articles (many award-winning) have appeared in numerous magazines and journals around the world. Susan is founder and president of *Health Unlimited*, a Los Angeles-based consulting firm dedicated to the advancement of human potential, wellness education, and motivation. In 1985, Susan was selected as one of ten "Healthy American Fitness Leaders" by the President's Council on Physical Fitness and Sports; other honorees include Jack LaLanne, Richard Simmons, Coach John Wooden, Senator Richard Lugar, gold-medalist John Nabers, George Allen, astronaut James Lovell, Jr., Kathy Smith, and Denise Austin. Susan also travels internationally as a wellness consultant and motivational speaker to community, corporate, and church groups. Her inspiring keynote presentations and workshop/retreats are often booked one to two years in advance. She appears regularly on radio and television talk shows, is the author of several books including *Choose to Live Peacefully*, and has produced her own audiocassette series *Celebrate Life!*, a series of seven tapes, as well as her latest cassette titled *How to Achieve Any Goal: The Magic of Creative Visualization/Living Your Vision*.

In her personal life, Susan combines reading, photography, and vegetarian cooking with hiking, ocean-swimming, jogging, weight training, cycling, kayaking, and horseback riding. Desiring more of a challenge, Susan Smith Jones completed a 100-mile run from Santa Barbara to Los Angeles and participates in triathlons. Susan (who has acquired the nickname of 'Sunny') resides in Brentwood, Los Angeles.

Other Celestial Arts books you may enjoy

☐ *Choose to Live Peacefully*
by Susan Smith Jones, Ph.D.
By nurturing our inner selves and living in personal peace, we can help to bring about global change. In this book, Susan Smith-Jones explores the many components of a peaceful, satisfying life—including exercise, nutrition, solitude, meditation, ritual, and environmental awareness—and shows how they can be linked to world peace.
$11.95 paper, 320 pages

☐ *The Ecology Cookbook*
by Nan Hosmer Pipstem and Judi Ohr
This "Earth Mother's Advisory" shows how nourishing ourselves properly can bring about peace of mind, spiritual awareness, planetary peace and healing, and a better environment. Includes recipes, herbal medicine, and ecological advice.
$11.95 paper, 144 pages

☐ *Staying Healthy with the Seasons*
by Elson Haas, M.D.
One of the most popular of the new health books, this is a blend of Eastern and Western medicines, nutrition, herbology, exercise, and preventive healthcare.
$11.95 paper, 252 pages

☐ *Staying Healthy with Nutrition*
by Elson Haas, M.D.
The long-awaited examination of how what we eat determines our health and wellbeing. Truly a complete reference work, it details every aspect of nutrition, from drinking water to medicinal foods to the latest biochemical research.
$24.95 paper, 1,200 pages

☐ *Instinctive Nutrition*
by Severen Schaeffer
Your body instinctively knows what nutrients it needs, and what you should eat to be healthy. This book shows how to overcome centuries of social conditioning and learn to listen to your body's real needs, for health, weight loss, and healing.
$8.95 paper, 224 pages

☐ *Love is Letting Go of Fear*
by Gerald Jampolsky, M.D.
One of the most popular New Age books ever. The lessons in this extremely popular little book, based on *A Course in Miracles*, will teach you to let go of fear and remember that our true essence is love. Includes daily exercises. Over 1,000,000 copies in print
$7.95 paper, or $9.95 cloth, 144 pages

☐ *Unlimit Your Life*
by James Fadiman, Ph.D.
How to assess and understand the factors holding you back in life, and then set concrete goals and start working towards attaining them in the most efective, life-affirming fashion.
$9.95 paper, 224 pages

☐ *The Common Book of Consciousness*
Revised Edition by Diana Saltoon

A beloved sourcebook, newly revised and updated for the 1990's. This guide to leading a whole and centered life shows how to use meditation, exercise, and nutrition to gain a higher consciousness and a full, balanced daily life.
$11.95 paper, 160 pages

☐ *Embrace Tiger, Return to Mountain*
by Chungliang Al Huang

The essence of the art of Tai Chi, presented by one of the world's foremost authorities, Huang's unique perspective is based in a deep yet playful understanding of Eastern tradition coupled with years of training in dance and martial arts.
$12.95 paper, 256 pages

☐ *Gentle Yoga*
by Lorna Bell, R.N. and Eudora Seyfer

This book is especially designed for people with arthritis, stroke damage, or multiple sclerosis, those in wheelchairs, or anyone who needs a gentle, practical way to improve their health through exercise. The book is spiralbound to stay open while you work and includes over 135 helpful illustrations.
$8.95 paper, 144 pages

☐ *Serenity* Second Edition
by Paul Reed

This book provides tools and strategies for confronting the fear of AIDS and gaining peace of mind, with emotional support and guidance for people with HIV, and their families, friends and caregivers. Leads readers from despair to action to hope.
$6.95 paper, 128 pages

☐ *Recovery from Addiction*
by John Finnegan and Daphne Grey

Alternative herbal and nutritional therapies for a wide range of addictions, from cigarettes to sugar to caffeine to hard drugs. Includes first-person accounts of how these treatments have worked for a variety of specific problems.
$9.95 paper, 192 pages

Available from your local bookstore, or order direct from the publisher. Please include $1.25 shipping & handling for the first book, and 50 cents for each additional book. California residents include local sales tax. Write for our free complete catalog of over 400 books and tapes.

Ship to:

Name _____

Address _____

City _____ State ____ Zip _____

Phone _____

Celestial Arts

Box 7327

Berkeley, CA 94707

For VISA or Mastercard orders

call (510) 845-8414